Care Homes for
Older People

Judith Torrington

E & FN SPON
An Imprint of Chapman & Hall
London · Weinheim · New York · Tokyo · Melbourne · Madras

**Published by E & FN Spon, an imprint of Chapman & Hall,
2–6 Boundary Row, London SE1 8HN, UK**

Chapman & Hall, 2–6 Boundary Row, London SE1 8HN, UK

Chapman & Hall GmbH, Pappelallee 3, 69469 Weinheim,
Germany

Chapman & Hall USA., 115 Fifth Avenue, New York
NY 10003, USA

Chapman & Hall Japan, ITP- Japan, Kyowa Building, 3F, 2–2–1
Hirakawacho, Chiyoda-ku, Tokyo 102, Japan

Chapman & Hall Australia, 102 Dodds Street, South Melbourne,
Victoria 3205, Australia

Chapman & Hall India, R. Seshadri, 32 Second Main Road, CIT
East, Madras 600 035, India

First edition 1996

© 1996 Judith Torrington

This book was commissioned by Maritz Vandenberg for
E & FN Spon

Typeset in 9/12 pt Univers Med by WestKey Limited, Falmouth,
Cornwall

Printed in Great Britain by The Alden Press, Oxford

ISBN   0 419 20120 3

A catalogue record for this book is available from the British
Library

Library of Congress Catalog Card Number: 96-67926

∞ Printed on acid-free text paper, manufactured in accordance
with ANSI/NISO Z39.48–1992 (Permanence of Paper).

Contents

vi **Acknowledgements**

vii **Introduction**

1 **1 The people**

1 1.1 The older person in
residential accommodation

25 1.2 Management structures

29 1.3 Regulators

30 1.4 The outside world

35 **2 Building design guide**

35 2.1 Anthropometrics

36 2.2 Activity and space requirements

77 2.3 Interior design

81 2.4 Services

85 2.5 Systems

90 2.6 Site

103 **3 Management of the
building process**

103 3.1 Statutory approvals and inspections

107 3.2 The building process

113 **4 Technical supplements**

114 TS1 List of suppliers

116 TS2 List of agencies concerned
with older people

117 TS3 List of dangerous and
poisonous plants

119 TS4 Initial briefing meeting agenda

120 TS5 Schedule of accommodation

122 TS6 Room data sheet

123 **Further reading**

125 **Index**

Acknowledgements

I am grateful to the people who have generously given me assistance and advice in the preparation of this book. I would especially like to thank the following:

- Audrey Marshall and the residents of Overdale for allowing me to photograph them
- Ruth Tregenza, my consultant
- Roger Coleman, Design Age, Royal College of Art; Richard Hollingbery, Visiting Policy Associate, Centre for Policy on Ageing, formerly Director, The Helen Hamlyn Foundation; Lady Sally Greengross, Age Concern; Sarah Langton-Lockton and Andrew Lacey, Centre for Accessible Environments; Dr R.T. McKinley, Horticultural Trades Association; Michael Manser, Manser Associates; Phippen Randall and Parkes, Architects; Nick Borrett, Design and Build Services Ltd; John Hannah, British Gypsum; Dr Harry Peake
- The University of Sheffield School of Architectural Studies
- Maritz Vandenberg, my editor
- Peter Tregenza and Hannah Swain for their help, support and encouragement

Introduction

Care homes for older people is a book for the commissioners of building work and their designers and builders. The profile of care providers in Great Britain is radically different from that of ten years ago; new buildings are being built, old ones upgraded, independent operators and trusts are taking over care responsibilities from the Local and Health Authorities. Care homes may offer day care and peripatetic services supporting older people in their own homes. Community Care legislation has brought change to everyone involved in the care of older people. Alongside the revolution in care provision are new techniques of procurement and production of buildings. This book deals with the design of care homes; it will chart the needs of the user, provide a detailed design guide and summarize the management of the building process.

Design for frail older people is a specialist area. Most of the built environment is so unsuitable for older people that they are unable to use it without assistance. The provision of residential buildings is highly regulated; the building users have specific needs. Methods of building procurement are evolving, so the personnel involved in the production of a building may alter over the life of a project. Patterns of care are changing. While there is no substitute for expertise and experience, this book aims to give a working knowledge of the area for those who become involved at whatever stage of the process.

The book is in three sections which can be used independently. The first part of the book concerns the building users and their needs. This includes staff, regulators and officials, relatives and visitors as well as the residents. User needs are identified from the perspective of an architect, not a medical or sociological expert, with a view to identifying the constraints on building design.

The second part is the design guide. This may be used as a desk top reference book. There is anthropometric information, space by space check lists which include illustrated space standards and items of commonly used equipment. There is a section on interior design dealing with colour, lighting and acoustics. Services and systems are covered where they are specific to the building type. The design guide concludes with the design of external spaces.

The last part of the book is concerned with project management. Statutory procedures and inspections which are required to register a care home are described, and finally the management of the building process including building procurement techniques is discussed.

There is a series of Technical Supplements at the end. These contain ancilliary information such as address lists which will be of use to some, but not all readers.

Working with the very old is a rewarding and privileged job. Care homes are inhabited by definition by people of resilience and fortitude, many of whom live with chronic disabilities. Perhaps the majority have experienced hardship, danger or war, the kind of difficulties unimaginable to the post-war generation largely responsible for their care. The challenge for designers and commissioners of buildings is to enable the people who will inhabit them to live out their lives in dignity with autonomy, comfort and choice, making the best of their remaining physical resources.

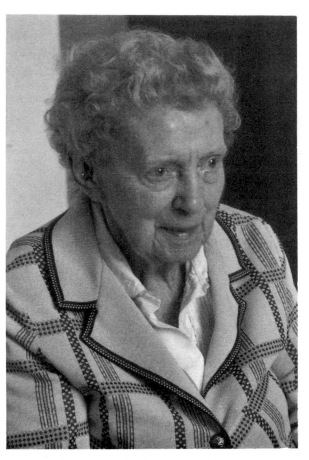
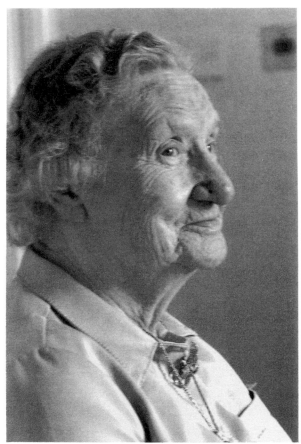
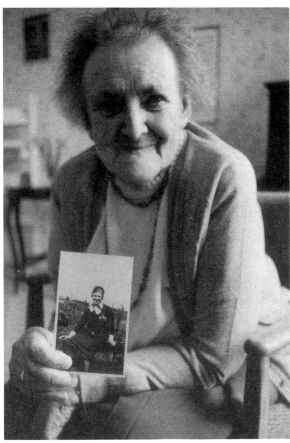
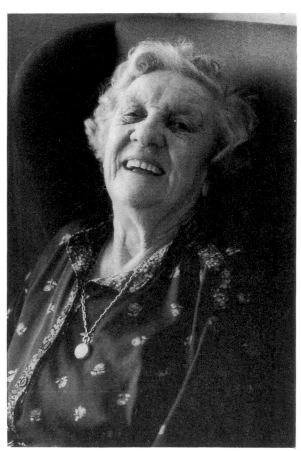

1 The people

1.1 The older person in residential accommodation

1.1.1 Statistics

The proportion of older people in the population has been growing steadily in Great Britain. Census data show that people aged 65 and over represented 13.2% of the population in 1971, 15% in 1981 and 15.8% in 1993. Current projections suggest that the rise in numbers of older people as compared with the rest of the population will continue well into the next century: in 2021 the figure is expected to be 19.4% rising to a peak of 24.6% in 2041. Within the 65+ age group the proportional growth in numbers of those aged 80 and over is even more marked. In 1971 2.3% of the population were over 80. By 1993 it was 3.9% and the numbers are predicted to rise steadily to 9.2% in 2051. As the proportion of older people grows the working population shrinks: the ratio of 'dependants', that is people over retirement age and under 16 to people of working age was 63 to 100 in 1992; it is expected to rise to more than 80 to 100 by the middle of the next century.

Most old people live out their lives in their own homes or with relatives in the community. The aim of current social policy is to support people living at home for as long as possible. There is however a significant number who need more support than can be provided in the community who move into residential care. The total numbers in homes for older people in Great Britain were around 198 000 in 1981 and 264 000 in 1993, representing 1–2% of the population over 65. Numbers of people moving into residential care were increasing proportionally between 1981 and 1993 as means-tested fee subsidy became universally available. The Community Care Act is expected to stem that tide. Now only those who are assessed as needing residential care can get financial support so people moving into homes tend to be older and frailer. The proportion of older people in care homes is likely to remain constant, at around 1.5% of the older population. It is unlikely that it will fall below this level, indeed the proportion of those needing residential care has not substantially altered since 1901. On the basis of current projections 369 000 care home places will be required by 2041.

Who are the people in residential care? What are their problems, hopes, limitations and expectations? Homes vary: some cater for all comers, others offer expert care for discrete groups. They range from specialist units for the severely mentally infirm, to hotel-style homes catering for the active older person, to family businesses in converted houses. Most registering authorities regard 40 places as the maximum acceptable size for a care home, with the result that many new buildings are built for that number. There is no typical care home for 40 residents. If such a home did exist and was representative of the entire care home population the following statements could be made about the residents:

- 13 would have established dementia.
- 28 would show mild/severe dementia.
- 13 would have no living spouse or children.
- 3 would have no relatives at all.
- 16 would suffer urinary incontinence.
- 16 would be male.
- 24 would be female.
- 1–2 would be aged 65–74, of whom 1 would be male and 1 female.
- 9 would be aged 75–84, of whom 4 would be male and 5 female.
- 30 would be aged 85+, of whom 11 would be male and 19 female.
- Most would have limited mobility.

Those who require residential care have difficulties of one kind or another which should be reflected in the design of buildings for them. Commissioners and designers of buildings come to the task with a specialist view and the design team will be made up of people with a wide range of skills. There is likely to be expertise in management, finance, health and social care, and design, although the actual building users are unlikely to be represented. Home managers are not often appointed at the briefing stage, and residents, their relatives or care assistants are rarely consulted which is a pity as building users can be valuable members of briefing teams.

Nursing and residential homes are designed to tight budgets and space is at a premium, but they are a relatively new building type and it is rare to visit one which does not suffer from design failures attributable to poor briefing decisions. The design defects listed below are common:

- bathrooms unused because of poor access to bath and lack of lifting aids;
- empty lounges too remote from the central areas for residents with limited mobility;
- overcrowded dayrooms where the only possible furniture arrangement is a circle of chairs round the perimeter of the room;
- residents eating off trays in lounges because dining rooms are too small or inaccessible;
- toilets near the main dayrooms with inadequate screening;
- insufficient space for staff to assist residents walking around the home, in bathrooms and toilets;
- identical or similar bedroom corridors which are disorientating to the staff as well as to residents;
- fire escape stairs used as storage areas (particularly for wheelchairs);
- a group of exiled smokers (residents and staff) round the service entrance;
- old people sitting in uncomfortable draughts at the front door in order to see something going on;
- en-suite toilets which do not get used because they are too small.

Experienced operators avoid these problems; it is quite clear that the more homes an organization has in management the better the briefing operation is.

1.1.2   Attitudes to old age

People in residential care are not the same. All they have incontrovertibly in common is old age but there are generalizations that can be made which should influence the design of the buildings for older people. Specific difficulties and their design implications are discussed later. Before we get into detail, society's attitude to ageing is worth consideration.

It is difficult to avoid sounding negative about old age. Inevitably ageing brings problems, and these are mostly related to health. Lists of the difficulties faced by older people give a pessimistic view of old age which is reinforced by practically everything written in the papers and seen on television. These discouraging attitudes inevitably rub off onto older people themselves, so to

The people

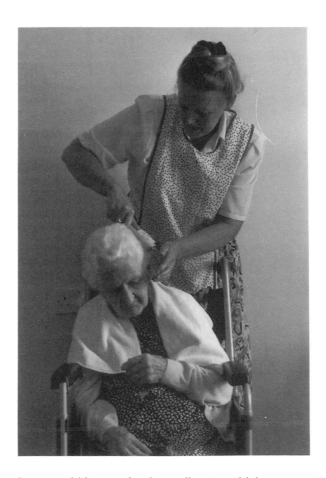

be very old is perceived as a disaster which we must somehow endure. This view does not obtain in other cultures, indeed it is peculiar to the West. Britain has one of the largest aged populations in relation to the whole population but there is a dismal perception of what it is to be old. The first responsibility of those concerned with designing for older people is to respect their clients. The building design can play a part in moulding attitudes to older people for good or ill.

A well-dressed, well turned out, manicured and coiffeured 90-year-old lady sitting in a well furnished room with flattering lighting is not treated in the same way, even by the professional carer, as one who is shabby and unkempt, sitting on a vinyl armchair with food stains on her clothing.

Individual rights can be eroded by institutional living. A rigid daily routine or the constraints imposed by the building should not be allowed to interfere with the resident's natural rights: to privacy, autonomy, freedom of sexuality, religious belief and practice, control of their own financial affairs, freedom to come and go and to take risks and to be treated with dignity.

The move into residential care, though initially traumatic can be a life-enhancing experience. Commonly the move happens after a crisis: a fall, an illness or the collapse of existing home care arrangements. An old person coming into a home could well have been struggling on a poor diet, with inadequate heating, high anxiety levels about money, home maintenance and a lonely life. A home provides company, both that of other residents, and perhaps more importantly with staff, warmth, good food and freedom from anxiety. A recent survey shows that 60% of people thought living in a home was better than they were expecting, with many people expressing the relief and satisfaction they felt in a safe and caring environment.

The issue of attitude is clearly as much to do with management standards as with the building, and some very good homes are run in rather inadequately designed premises. Some principles which should influence the design of new buildings are listed below.

- The building is the resident's home; others just work there. Personal and semi-private territory needs to be defined and respected.
- The building should facilitate good personal presentation of the residents. Clothes' laundering and ironing, hairdressing and grooming activities must be well catered for.
- Lighting should be designed to flatter residents as well as fulfilling functional requirements.
- Residents should never be seen in an undignified situation. Screening of bathing and toilet areas is essential.
- Supervision should be unobtrusive. Staff access and supervision should not be at the expense of comfortable sitting areas.

1.1.3 Challenges of ageing

The most common problems that may affect the design of buildings for old people are discussed below. They need to be understood as the building can magnify or minimize the difficulties. The aim is to make the very best of the resources the old person has. A resident should not have to battle to open her bedroom door against a strong sprung door closer; that energy could be used to take a turn around the garden. To be old is to acquire a tolerance of disabilities which may be quite minor when they first appear. One 98-year-old woman, when asked how she was said 'I can't see very well, and I'm pretty deaf now and I can't walk much but I'm all right in myself.'

1.1.4 The ageing body

Many of the problems faced by the people who live in care homes are caused not by illness but the natural gradual degeneration of the body. It is the tough old survivors who represent the bulk of the care home population. The killing diseases hit a younger age group. Deaths from heart disease and cancer mainly affect people aged between 65 and 74 and strokes and respiratory illness tend to occur between the ages of 75 and 85.

In very old age the body tends to slow down and seize up. The response to injury and to external stimulus is slow, so someone may lean on a hot radiator long enough to sustain burns before they realize that it is hot. The digestive function loses efficiency. The kidneys and bladder do not work so well as formerly, so old people may need to urinate more frequently than others. Constipation is a common problem, and a good diet is as important for the very old as it is for the very young. The skin becomes fragile and easily injured and slow to heal; bed sores and ulcers are common. Many old people do not have the strength to operate commonly specified items of ironmongery. Old people are not very agile and lose some sense of balance. They also can suffer short unpredictable fainting fits; they are in danger of and fear falling. Temperature extremes are not well tolerated. In hot climates the heat waves kill the old; in Great Britain hypothermia is more common.

There is an increased vulnerability to certain illnesses, like pneumonia and food poisoning which is why the hygiene standards and precautions against infections such as Legionnaire's disease are so stringent.

Most of the built environment is actually unusable by frail older people. Some key issues which will affect design are:

Building layout
- Measures to reduce the risk of cross infection are likely to be required.

Access and mobility
- Short travel distances for residents are important.

Interior detailed design
- Door closers and ironmongery should not restrict resident's ability to get around. Automatic hold open devices may be required.
- Main routes will need handrails.

- Furniture and fittings need to be suitable for older people.
- Areas of the building and circulation routes should be easy to identify.

Environment

- Constant temperatures are required. Most authorities now insist on approving contingency plans for providing heating in the event of power failure.
- Hot pipes and heaters must be protected. Maximum acceptable surface temperature is 43°C.
- The ability to control temperature and sunlight penetration, particularly in bedrooms and sitting rooms, is important to residents.

Services

- Hot water system should be designed to prevent infection with Legionnaire's disease.

1.1.5 Mobility

Most old people in residential care are severely restricted in their mobility. The only group to whom this may not apply are the dementia sufferers who may be very active. There are various reasons for mobility restriction. Osteo-porosis is very common, especially in old women. Several residents may have suffered broken limbs, and will fear falling again. The disease particularly affects the spine and the weight-bearing joints in the legs leading to limited and painful movement. Stroke or hemiplegia can cause paralysis of one side of the body. This can affect either side so aids and supports need to be symmetrical.

In a typical 40-bed home there may be five active residents, 20 walking around but slowly, needing support from handrails, staff or walking aids, 10 moved around in wheelchairs and five totally inactive, perhaps because of illness. Of the 25 walkers a high proportion will have suffered a distressing fall.

The active older resident

This group comprises those who can make their way around the home unaided by staff, albeit with some difficulty. They are likely to be in the minority.

Access to all parts of the home, inside and out is essential if choice is to have any meaning for the individual resident. Choice is already severely limited by the fact of living in an institution, however well managed; residents live in an environment where many things are decided for them, from the decor to the menus. Remaining choices like where to sit and how to spend the day should be actively promoted. Choices can be as severely restricted by the physical nature of the surroundings as by the norms of custom and habit which settle like lead on any institution.

The active resident will be able to walk, perhaps with the aid of a walking frame or stick. Walking may be a slow shuffle; the feet may drag along the ground or there may be a pronounced limp. Additional supports will be in constant use. Life will be complicated by the need to carry things around – you cannot leave your knitting and your book, your crochet rug and your handbag by your chair like you do at home, they all go with you. The route from the bedroom to the dayroom can be an obstacle course for an unsteady person on a Zimmer frame hung about like a Christmas tree with possessions. The design aim should be to eliminate or minimize the real obstacles and mitigate the psychological ones.

Assisted walkers

There could be around 40% of residents who will be helped around by staff, either in walking or in wheelchairs.

It is harder to ensure that this group can choose how or where to spend their time. The tendency is for these residents to be found in the same place every day, that place being the main day room nearest the dining room. This arrangement may be perfectly satisfactory to the person concerned but it is important that the building does not limit choice. A variety of sitting areas

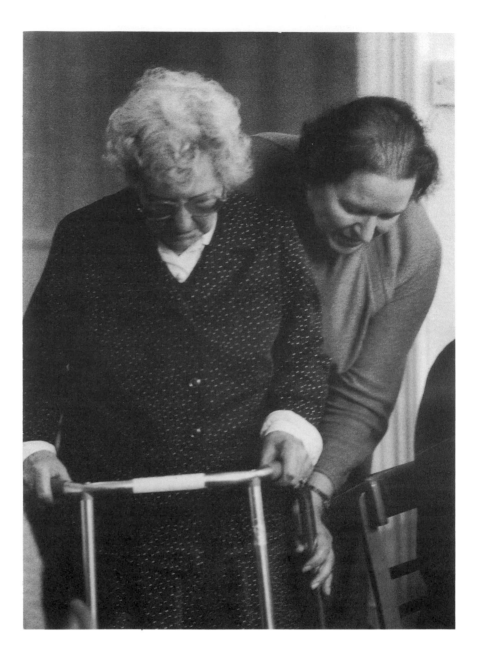

should be available, some quiet, some bustling, with or without television. Small quiet rooms are desirable but they will be underused if they are remote. Room shapes should not preclude different furniture arrangements. The dreary circle of chairs which is so common in care homes is often the only practical way to arrange the room.

Room-bound residents

Some people are not joiners and may prefer to stay in their own rooms at least some of the time. They may not like the society of other residents or they may be unable to communicate usefully with them. Bedrooms are designed down to size. The design of this room, the only private space for the individual in the home, is a challenge in 10–12 m^2. The bedroom should also function as a sitting room, with a good sitting position. It will be used to entertain visitors.

Residents in bed

Inevitably from time to time there will be residents confined to bed because of illness or extreme weakness. Good access is required around the bed for nursing and for visitors, and it should be possible for a bed-bound person to get a view out of the window.

The restricted mobility of residents is perhaps the major influence on building design. A summary of the points to be considered follows:

The people

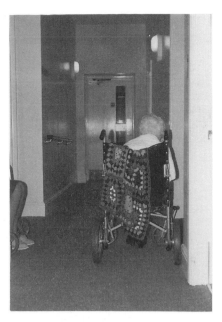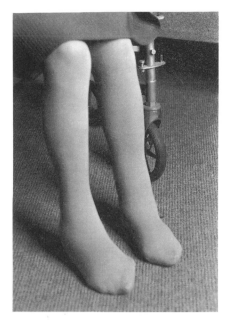

Building layout

- Changes in level are best avoided. If this is not possible ramps will be required inside and outside the building:

     maximum ramp gradient is 1 in 12;

     maximum ramp length for a 1 in 12 to 1 in 15 slope is 5 metres;

     maximum ramp length for a 1 in 15 to 1 in 20 slope is 10 metres.

- Is there a good route to a car or ambulance at the front door?
- Room location and travel distance. The distance each resident has to move daily is far greater than they have been used to in a domestic house and is often seen as daunting. Is the distance from bedroom to any area visited daily greater than 40 metres?
- Is the end destination visible or are there long dark corridors shut off by fire doors? How many doors have to be negotiated on the main routes? The journey will not seem so arduous if the destination can be seen or if there is some incident, a window or a resting place on the way.
- Lift location. Lifts are very heavily used and should be in the location chosen to minimize travel distances. This means in the middle. Handrails should be fitted in lifts.
- Is there immediate straightforward access to the toilets from all lounges and dining rooms?
- Small lounges, if provided, give an opportunity for quieter areas away from the crowd and the television, and are good for entertaining visitors but they will not be used unless they are accessible from the other areas where residents spend the day. The family group-living concept adopted in some homes with day areas for each group means travel distances are minimized, although additional staff may be needed.
- Is there something interesting to look at through the windows of the dayrooms?
- Does the size or shape of any room preclude alternative furniture arrangements or wheelchair access?
- Is wheelchair storage available near to where it will be required?
- Is the route to outside sitting areas direct, and is it easy to get back inside again?
- Are the toilets accessible from the outside sitting areas?
- Can a person confined to bed still see a good view through the window?
- Is there space for visitors in the bedrooms?
- Is the television or radio within reach of the bedroom chair?
- Access around the bed must be good from all sides.

Access and mobility

- Two people in wheelchairs or walking with frames should be able to pass in the corridors.

- All doors used by residents should be wide enough for wheelchairs.
- Is it necessary to open heavy doors on the main routes? Has the provision of magnetic hold open devices linked to the fire alarm been considered on the doors in the main circulation routes?
- Is it possible to go outside with a wheelchair through all doors?
- Does the handrail continue outside?
- Is there some destination like a seat in easy reach?
- Are the thresholds flush?
- Are the pavings level and smooth or are there drainage channels or gaps in which walking frame legs or walking sticks could stick?

Interior detailed design

- Handrails will be in constant use. Some older people will only be able to use one side for support, so a handrail on only one side of a corridor will get them where they are going but not back. Breaks in handrails often occur, inevitably at doors but also past sitting areas in corridors or at windows. These should be avoided if possible. Handrails should not be sited over unprotected heaters and should not lead people to something they might bump into (for instance a fire alarm panel with sharp edges mounted on a wall above the handrail). Handrails are expensive and often omitted as late budget cuts; savings should be considered in relation to the time taken by staff helping residents round the building who may otherwise be able to manage alone. Brackets need to be strong and well fixed – handrails get very heavy use.
- Are the doors wide enough for wheelchairs or for staff walking alongside residents?
- Everything approximately at handrail height will be used for support, whether it is a towel rail or a heater cover and must be strongly fixed and suitable to be grasped.
- Are the floor finishes continuous?
- Are floor finishes suitable for wheels; are they self cleansing by entrance doors?
- Is there somewhere to put things in reach of the armchair in the bedroom? Telephone, knitting, letters, photographs, the somewhat dwindling pile of possessions, all connect the resident to life.
- Is there room for a footstool in the bedroom?

Environment

- Do glazing bars obstruct the view through the windows?

Services

- Hot water pipes and heating units must be routed where they will not be touched.
- Is the nurse call button within reach of sitting positions in unsupervised rooms?

1.1.6 Eyesight

People's eyesight alters with age. The lens becomes inflexible and the eye muscles lose their ability to shorten the focal length with the result that in old age the focus becomes fixed eventually at infinity. Short sighted people benefit from this process and they may find improvements in vision as they get older, but most people will find some deterioration. Visual performance is altered in a number of ways which are significant when it comes to designing successful environments for old people.

Light quantity and quality

Less light reaches the retina, so more light is needed for visual tasks. To achieve a similar visual performance an older person can need as much as three times as much light as a 20-year-old. Apart from the natural ageing process there are diseases of the eye which affect older people, such as glaucoma and cataract, both treatable conditions in the short term but which ultimately tend to lead to loss of vision. There needs to be sufficient light, particularly to draw attention to hazards like changes in level. The quality of the lighting is of equal importance; lighting levels should be high, but glare free. Light needs to be well directed.

Glare	There is a scattering of light within the eye which increases sensitivity to glare. The muscles of the eye are slow to adjust, so going from a dark space to a light one can cause temporary blindness. Shiny surfaces should be avoided.
Colour vision	The lens thickens and yellows so that colour vision is affected; blues and greens are not so easily distinguished as reds and yellows.
Orientation	There may be loss of peripheral vision, which has an important function of detecting movement and spatial awareness, making orientation more difficult. The ability to judge depth may be impaired partly because of loss of the ability to distinguish receding colours, and partly because of the dazzling effect of contrasting light and darkness.

For detail design requirements see section 2.3.1 Colour and light.

1.1.7 Hearing

As with eyesight there is a natural deterioration in hearing due to ageing. The auditory nerve loses efficiency as we get older, a condition known medically as presbycusis. This is likely to affect every resident in the home to some degree. A further cause of deafness in older people is cortical deafness due to a defect in the brain centres, and if there are men present who served in the second world war, they may have been exposed to very loud noise without protection which has a similar effect on hearing as presbycusis. The condition causes loss of ability to hear high frequency sounds but the capacity to hear loud noises is not affected. Hearing loss is at low sound levels, so while soft speech may be inaudible shouting is uncomfortable to the hearer, which is why people so often say 'There's no need to shout, I'm not deaf' when a remark is repeated rather louder than before.

Since virtually all the residents will have some hearing loss it is important that the acoustic environment is as good as possible with an emphasis on magnifying high frequency sounds, minimizing background noise and aiming at a dead acoustic rather than long reverberation times. A good acoustic environment is a precious commodity for people with poor hearing.

Acoustic design is discussed in more detail in section 2.3.2.

1.1.8 Manual dexterity

Restricted movement in the hands causing discomfort or severe pain is relatively common in older people.

Some causes are rheumatoid arthritis, Parkinson's disease, or stroke leading to partial paralysis. Designers and commissioners of buildings can get some idea of the problems, if not the pain, by wearing a thick pair of leather gloves for a day.

All parts of the building which are handled by residents should be designed for easy manipulation. Areas needing attention are listed below.

Restricted hand movement

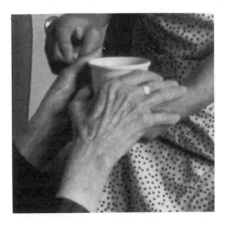 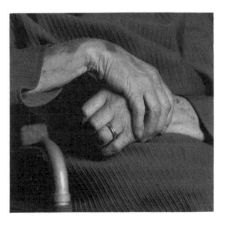

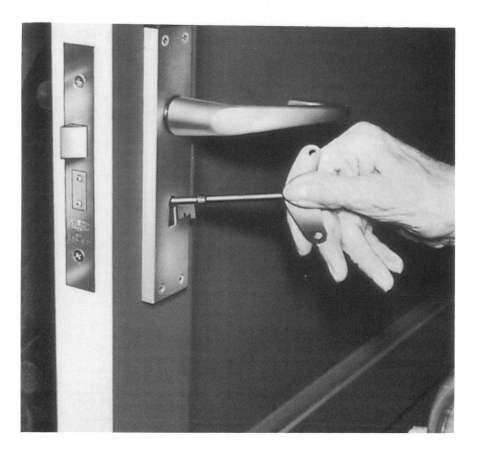

- Ironmongery, including any on built-in furniture needs to be selected with care. Lever and D handles are preferred to knobs in any form. Sharp edges and stiff action should be avoided. Snibs need to be large. Some suppliers design door furniture specifically for older people, see Technical Supplement 1 for a list.
- Sanitary fittings should be selected with care. Lever taps are preferred to cross top, which are better than plastic knobs which offer no resistance to turning.
- Electric switches should be rocker type, with the switches on the outside of double sockets.
- Nurse call points and extension leads should be easy to handle.
- Fitting out is not covered in this book, but the same principles apply to the selection of cutlery etc.

1.1.9 Incontinence

Incontinence is the inability to control the reflex emptying of the bladder or rectum due to loss of co-ordination of the nervous system, or through damage to the bladder or rectum caused by disease, childbirth or accident. The onset of incontinence may be the straw that breaks the camel's back as far as home carers are concerned, and is often the reason for admission to a residential institution. Estimates of the numbers of sufferers vary: a residential home may have 40% occasionally incontinent residents while in long-stay hospital care there could be up to 70%. Good management routines can make a significant impact on these numbers.

Incontinence can cause great grief to the sufferer who may find the state almost unbearable. When it is apparent that someone is incontinent it has an effect on the attitude of other people to that person, be they visitors, relations or even professional carers. Because it is such a common condition in care homes the staff can become blasé about it and treat the condition with robust good humour which can deepen the distress of the sufferer.

The management of incontinence is one of the main concerns of the day-to-day running of a home. Those which fail to deal with incontinence as a management issue smell bad. The policy adopted needs to be addressed in some detail at the briefing stage. A poor or incomplete understanding of the problem can make a carefully furnished and beautifully decorated home seem like a Victorian workhouse; there is nothing so institutional as a smell.

Each resident will be assessed regularly. Some people can be cured of incontinence, others can benefit from good management of the condition. Techniques used are control of diet, a routine of going to the toilet, exercises and continence aids. Residents will be taken to the toilet regularly by the care staff. The toilets adjacent to the day areas will be the most heavily used. This is a time-consuming tedious routine in a busy day and care staff can and do become insensitive to the need to maintain the dignity and privacy of residents. Toilets should be designed to screen users from general view even if staff do leave the doors open. The toilets should be pleasant for the residents to use; they are also a working area for staff who need good access to help residents, preferably on each side of the pan. Continence aids should be stored conveniently near and there should be facilities for washing and changing people if necessary. Drains need to be designed for good rodding access. Incontinence pads and even underwear quite frequently get flushed away.

However well managed a home is, accidents will inevitably happen. Accidental soiling needs to be dealt with as soon as possible, and at least within a stated time objective of less than 20 minutes; the resident should be washed or showered and changed and the soiling cleaned before stains and smells can become established within the fabric of the building. Good ventilation is essential.

The building design needs to take account of the following points:

Building layout

- Toilets are needed adjacent to day rooms and dining rooms where they will be used in relays by one or two care staff to each resident. It is better to have a space each side of the pan for staff to assist.
- Toilets need to be screened from view of the main circulation routes to maintain dignity and privacy. It is better if screening is achieved by room layout rather than doors which may be propped open by busy staff.
- Toilets in or near bedrooms will be used in the morning and at night. Around 75% of residents need assistance, so if en-suite toilets do not have space for a helper they will not be used.
- Sufficient storage for incontinence pads, bedpans and urine bottles will be required, preferably in the sluice in each bedroom group and convenient for the toilets near the dayrooms.
- Cleaners' stores will be required within good reach of all areas with water supply, bucket sink and space for upright floor cleaners.

Interior detailed design

- Floor finishes, fabrics, chair covers etc., must be suitable for cleaning. There is a list of suppliers of suitable carpets in Technical Supplement 1. Toilets should be easy to clean but should preferably not be too clinical in appearance.

Environment

- Toilets need to be warm, light and comfortable.
- Good ventilation, preferably both mechanical and natural is important.

Services

- Disposal of incontinence pads will block the drains. Good access for rodding and simple drainage layouts are essential.

1.1.10 Dementia; the confused older person

For most people intellectual function does not significantly diminish with age; small loss of brain cell efficiency is compensated for by experience. It is reasonable to assume that someone in a residential home may have stiff joints, diminished eyesight and poor hearing but not that there will be any impairment in intellect. There is, however, a group of people who do suffer serious mental impairment in old age as a result of disease or damage to the brain, who can be described as suffering brain failure, otherwise known as dementia. People with dementia suffer progressive loss of brain function. Such is the nature of their disability that they are more likely than the general population to require residential care.

The understanding of dementia is the subject of much current and recent research. Only the most broad description of the condition is attempted here. There does appear to be a consensus that sensitive design can profoundly influence the well-being of the confused person and designers and commissioners of buildings for this group need a working knowledge of the nature of dementia.

Statistics of dementia

A true statistical picture of the incidence of dementia in the population cannot be obtained. The onset of dementia is often unrecognized, and there are a large number who have the condition undiagnosed. It has been suggested that 1% of the 65–74 age group and 10% of those over 75 suffer from dementia. In 1991 there were approximately 480 000 people with the condition with numbers predicted to rise steadily to 600 000 by 2025.

A very rough estimate of numbers of people suffering from dementia at present would indicate that between 30 and 40% are in institutional care, and that these are distributed unevenly among the residential institutions in approximately the following ratios:

- private homes   30%
- local authority homes 40%
- NHS homes   60%

Assuming a home size of 40 residents on the basis of these figures, private homes would have 12 dementia sufferers, local authority old persons' homes would have 16 and NHS homes 24. These figures are borne out by observation; there are specialist units for people suffering from severe dementia, but there are also significant numbers of confused older people in most nursing and residential homes.

So all residential homes will care from time to time for confused people, and some will be designed specifically for dementia sufferers.

The nature of dementia

This is a designer's attempt to interpret a condition and to highlight the implications of that condition for the built environment.

Dementia is a condition caused by changes within the brain. The changes can be in the chemistry of the brain tissue, as in Alzheimer's disease or in the physical structure caused by numerous small haemorrhages like a number of small strokes. There are other possible causes such as Huntington's chorea or drug toxicity. Not all dementias are untreatable so it is important to have a good diagnosis of the cause which is the destruction of the connections between nerve cells. The process is usually progressive and irreversible but good management and nursing techniques can greatly improve the quality of life of the sufferer and may delay the progress of the disease. Central to the condition, unlike other forms of mental handicap or impairment, is the loss of personality of the sufferer.

The causes of brain nerve destruction are not known. The older you get the higher your chances of getting the disease. More women develop it than men. The condition is not related to socio-economics; the rich suffer as well as the poor. There are hereditary factors, and sometimes, though not necessarily, it can occur in families with one sibling succumbing after another. In such families the youngest member has a big burden of care and some fear for their own future.

Progress of the disease

The onset of dementia can be in middle age, though mostly it affects people over 65. In the early stages there is forgetfulness and memory failure. People cannot recall a name or a word. Such events usually go unremarked; they are common in most people and it is only when the condition becomes established and diagnosed that the history of its development is constructed. Memory lapses increase and can be very frustrating leading to outbursts of anger, aggression and also depression as the mildly impaired sufferer becomes conscious of failing powers. The losses may cause deliberate self limitation. If tests are carried out in the early stages they will show learning impairment and poor memory test performance; people cannot retrieve data from memory and the ability to acquire new data and store it is limited. This is a difficult time for relatives; household and financial management tasks can become a great burden to the sufferer and there may be outbursts of apparently inappropriate anger and paranoia.

When the condition becomes established the problem is more likely to be acknowledged and diagnosed. Memory and learning become disconnected. People find themselves in rooms with no idea of why they went there. Kettles get put on and forgotten, the gas turned on and not ignited, meals put out and not eaten. Knowledge of and interest in the outside world diminishes, and also the personal world of family and friends. There can be 'holes' in the memory: people or things may not be recognized. The dementia sufferer lives in the present moment.

Around a third of the mildly impaired suffer serious depression as a result of their condition. Some show signs of anxiety and aggression, others manifest an emotional indifference. The depression, anxiety and aggression diminish as the disease progresses and the sufferer becomes more disconnected from life.

Established dementia

As the disease progresses memory failures become very marked. There is an inability to recognize objects, for example that a sleeve is something you put your arm into. Changes in floor finish can be confused with a step. People are not able to recognize themselves in a mirror. There is disengagement from events in the world, then friends and family. The ability to dress, eat or keep clean, indeed the whole concept of self is lost. Many of the confused are restless, particularly those who have led an active life. They wander about, or perform self-imposed tasks over and over again. Many are active and physically fit, capable of covering considerable distances in their travels. There may be logic to be discerned from the activities being performed; people will get up and go to a previous work place, but they may get lost on the way. A former tradesman may go to 'work' on the plumbing installation (many of the activities can be destructive to the building fabric). Individuals have their own timetables which are at odds with the rest of the world; they will get up and dress in the middle of the night and want meals at times which may not suit institutions.

People can become disorientated in time of life as well as time of day. They may have one-sided conversations with someone long dead, such as their mother. When confronted with the truth they may confabulate (deny they were doing it) or say they were talking to someone in the next room. The disorientations in time and space can cause frustration and anger.

Someone with dementia may become more dependant on others for personal care: 40%–50% of people with established dementia are incontinent two or three times a week and a further 20% are occasionally incontinent. The onset of incontinence varies with the individual and can be influenced both by physical loss of function and regime. The ability to dress and clean oneself can disappear.

210 Knights Hill: a continuing care unit for elderly and severely mentally impaired residents designed by Manser Associates, 1991–1992. Planned for small family groups, the top lit central street helps residents to locate themselves and staff to supervise unobtrusively. Corridor lengths are kept to a minimum. Planning and site restrictions have compressed the building site so that the dayrooms have less good access to outside light and view than intended and the central spaces are artificially lit to compensate. There is easy access to a secure garden for the residents to wander in

Right. Plan

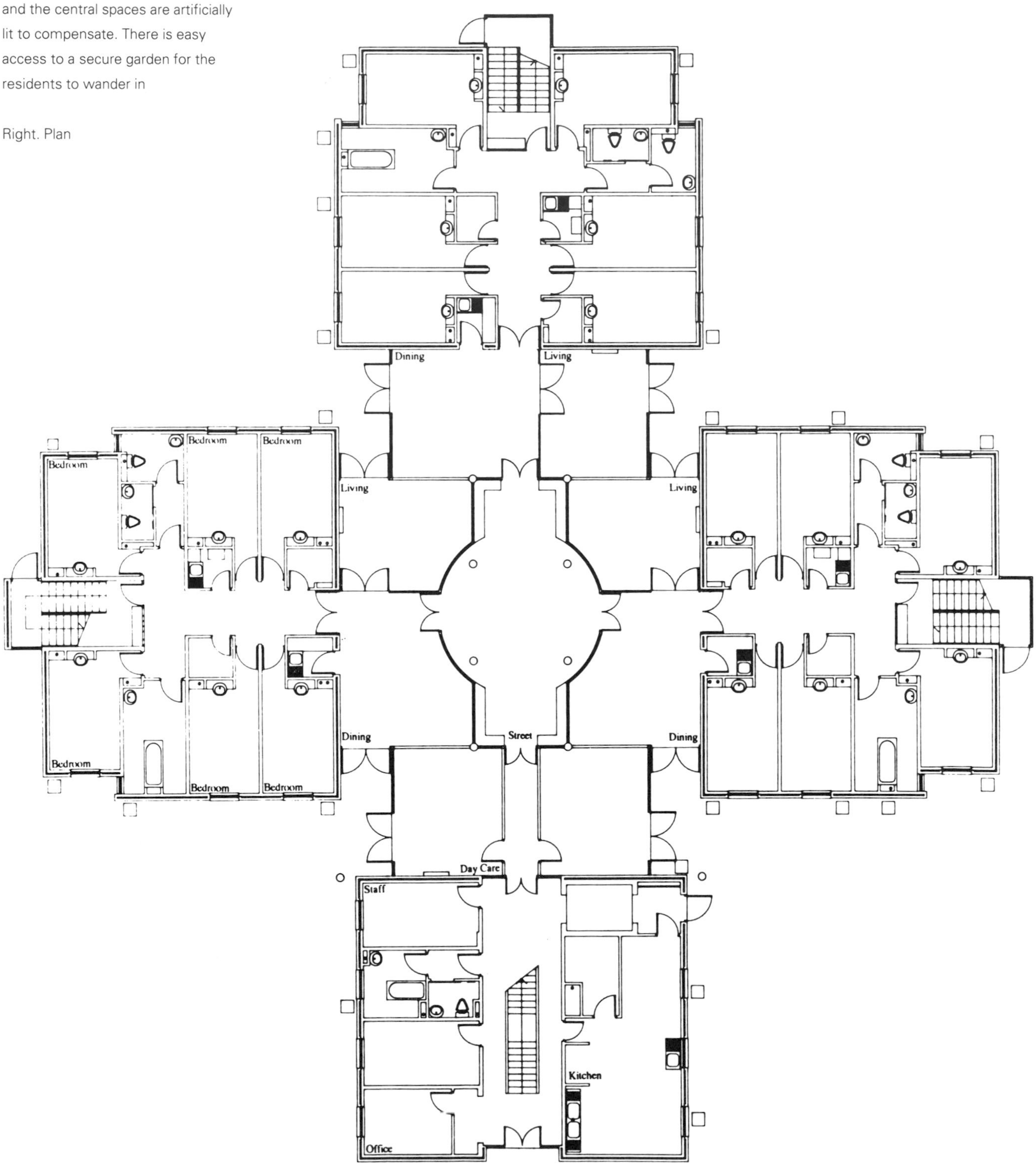

Dining

Living

Bedroom

Bedroom

Bedroom

Living

Living

Bedroom

Bedroom

Bedroom

Dining

Street

Dining

Day Care

Staff

Office

Kitchen

The people

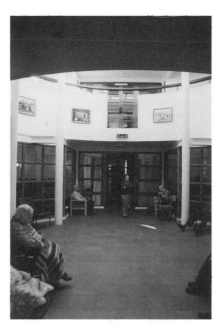 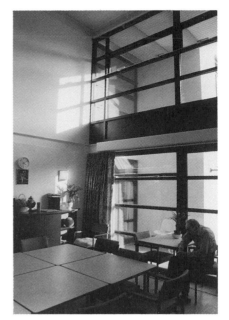

Disinhibition is a symptom of dementia. This leads to shouting, swearing, sexual display and advances made indiscriminately which can cause embarrassment to others. A confused lady may find hair washing or bathing unbearable, perhaps because of a fear of burning or drowning and will loudly proclaim the fact if anyone tries to perform either task.

Relationships can be disrupted; a demented person can reject a long-suffering partner or carer in favour of a formerly absent relation or a casual acquaintance.

Severe dementia

In the final stages of the disease the sufferer is in a burnt-out state with minimal voluntary activity. People become physically very frail, some will have other diseases of old age like osteoporosis in addition to their dementia. There can be complete loss of language, inability to speak as well as understand, or endless repetition of words or sentences. People may die from heart, liver or other organ failure, without warning, or there may be a time of extreme weakness when the sufferer is hardly able to move. At this stage people require a high degree of nursing care and skill.

Design for dementia

What is the appropriate architecture for the shattered and disintegrating mind? Much of the advice available is necessarily built on conjecture as it is not possible to get feed back from the sufferers themselves. Attempts have been made to evaluate the effect of different environments on those suffering dementia, but since no buildings are directly comparable, and no two groups of confused people are passing through the same stage of the disease at the same time this remains more of an art than a science.

People with dementia are accommodated in all kinds of buildings. There are the specialist units run by or for Health Authorities. These range from the characteristic Nightingale Wards with two dozen beds on either side of a nurse station and a dayroom, to new purpose-built developments, sometimes contracted out to independent operators. The housing associations provision for this group tend to be based on domestic house scale units, typically a group of linked bungalows. Some housing associations are very active in this field, with care sections managing a portfolio of care homes. There are homes run by Local Authorities or independent operators for the mentally infirm. All types of specialist accommodation tend to have additional input of care from the NHS, voluntary bodies or Local Authorities.

In addition to the buildings dedicated to the care of the mentally infirm are non-specialist nursing and residential homes in the public, private and voluntary sector, all of which from time to time are likely to house some confused people, and there are large numbers of people being cared for by relatives in their own homes. The specialist units sometimes offer respite care and day centres to people who live in the community and it is likely that this kind of provision will increase.

Most of the providers of homes for the demented have well developed sets of principles on which their buildings are designed. There are differing views and approaches, and since the philosophy will profoundly influence the form of the building it is important that the aims of a particular project are clearly stated at the outset.

Size and organization

Experts in the field advocate small homes for 30 or at the most 40 residents organized in family groups. The advice is reflected in the guidelines of many of the Health Authorities and Social Services Departments and a limit of 40 residents per home is often imposed. Size restrictions are opposed by many service providers for economic reasons. There is no doubt that larger homes are more cost effective; they make better use of laundry and kitchen facilities; more flexible staffing arrangements are possible, and a greater range of services can be provided. The cost of providing residential care in a specialist unit is very high, perhaps twice the cost of a place in a typical residential home. The numbers of people needing this kind of care are rising; it seems inevitable that the economic arguments will win the day and that nursing and residential homes will cater for increasing numbers. Ingenious design solutions are required to ensure confused residents can feel at home in big complicated buildings.

The most successful therapies for dementia sufferers are based on reinforcement of the familiar. Some people react very badly to relocation, and in any case few people are used to living with large numbers of others. Many of the successful homes for dementia sufferers are based on small self-contained family groups, ideally of eight people, but up to 13 have been adopted. The groups have discrete living and sleeping areas and live as a self-contained unit, with staff dedicated to their care. This is not the cheapest option: staff costs take up between 60% and 70% of the annual budget of a residential institution, and a building form which demands one additional staff member will have an impact on the fee for each resident.

It is common practice to segregate groups according to the severity of their condition. It can be distressing for someone with dementia to be with people in a more advanced stage of the disease, and in an all-purpose home the confused residents may trouble the others. Consideration may be given to the provision of a segregated area for a small group of residents. At least some separate sitting areas are desirable so that one or two disturbed and disturbing people can be parted from the rest. These should be located where they can be supervised without the need for additional staff or they will not be used.

A safe environment

People with dementia behave in a way which involves risk to themselves and to others. Many of those in residential care are there because their families can no longer cope with the dangers of living with the demented. Buildings for confused people need to be safe, but they should also respect the freedom of the individual. The safest environment is a big open hospital ward with everyone sitting in one space under the eye of the nursing sister within locked doors. The therapeutic value of such an environment is not high. Perhaps the greatest area of disagreement between different providers is the view that is taken on risk versus security. Regimes which give residents the most freedom and autonomy do so in the knowledge that they have to accept a higher degree of risk than those where the residents are highly supervised and monitored.

The liberal approach is elegantly summed up in a briefing document prepared by Guys Hospital and Lewisham NHS Trust for a project to house people with dementia in ordinary houses, called the Domus. The five assumptions of the Domus philosophy (HMSO, 1992) are:

1 The Domus is for dementia.
2 Unavoidable consequences of dementia are to be accommodated rather than 'solved', as opposed to avoidable (or minimizable) consequences which should be attended to with vigour.
3 Quality of life equals trouble and strife.
4 Look after the staff and the staff will look after the clients.
5 Emotional needs may take precedence over physical needs.

Essentially the Domus is a permanent home: residents do as much for themselves as possible even if this entails risk and untidiness, bedrooms are personal, there are set mealtimes but food is available all the time, bedtimes and rising times are flexible, there is a wide range of activities, and nursing needs will not necessarily dominate. The well-being of the staff is seen as essential to the success of the Domus and support for the staff is provided by means of training and development programmes and good on-site staff accommodation.

At the other end of the spectrum are the providers who see the provision of a safe and secure environment as one of their highest priorities. There is often pressure from relatives of confused people whose overriding concern is that their own should not come to harm. Such groups may object to the replacing of the old hospital wards with single-room accommodation because of fears that people may fall out of bed at night unseen. The challenge is to enable staff to observe and supervise residents without infringing the liberty and dignity of the individual.

The attitude towards risk needs to be addressed at the outset; it has consequences for all aspects of the building design, from choice of ironmongery to design of landscape and enclosure. The risks to be taken need to be clearly defined; clearly the building must be safe for a confused resident in the sense that there are no exposed heating pipes or unexpected steps. A demented resident should not impose any threat to other residents. The aim is to avoid causing unnecessary frustration and distress to the demented person by accommodating the patterns of behaviour which are the inevitable consequences of the condition where it is possible to do so. Management regime, staff attitudes and training contribute to this objective, and the physical environment should enable rather than thwart the user. Disturbed timetables will entail sleeping and eating to happen at odd times, and the bedroom, kitchen and dining arrangements should not preclude this. Wandering routes through the building and the gardens can be planned. The best routes are those which have incidents along the way with interesting stopping places where things happen, such as the entrance, a fountain in the garden, a place to watch the activities in the street, or deliveries to the kitchen.

Good visibility inside the building is essential. Staff need to be able to see what is happening but preferably in a discreet way. Day-time supervision is best achieved by clear open areas, divided by low partitions or screens. Night-time supervision can be more difficult. Some residents are likely to be awake at night, indeed they may be having their 'day'. Where the accommodation is in single rooms the staff need to know that all is well within the room; people can fall out of bed or get up and have a battle with the wash basin and may do much damage to themselves and the building fabric before anyone finds out.

Limitations of access for the confused resident need to defined at an early stage. There may be no restrictions at all or there may be a requirement to prevent or discourage access to the surrounding neighbourhood and to rooms within the home which could impose risks to the health or safety of the resident. Rooms which will have restricted access are those containing drugs and clinical supplies, those containing confidential records, kitchens, laundries, sluices, boiler rooms, electrical switchgear rooms and lift motor rooms. Access can be restricted by various techniques. Some homes will rely on care assistants and other staff to gently distract anyone bent on going into the no-go areas, others will use technology. Passive techniques can be effective and cause less frustration to residents than physical restrictions. People with dementia live essentially in the here and now, so they are easily distracted. A mirror fixed to the inside of a door seems to stop wanderers in their tracks, either because they think someone is approaching them, or they may become fascinated by their reflection and lose the intention of walking away. The door may also be locked but the resident will be saved from the frustration of finding themselves locked in or out.

An early decision is required on the degree of security of the site. A driveway will be needed for parking and service and ambulance vehicles and it is unlikely to be gated, or if it is the gates will often be open. The rest of the site will therefore be accessible unless it is fenced off. The options are to keep the site open, to fence off the garden area or to fence off a small area for use by confused people who are at risk of wandering away and getting lost. If the object is containment of the wanderers, gates will need to be openable from the outside and it is important to check that all the fire escape doors to the building open inside the enclosure, or, if not, that appropriate ironmongery or alarms are fitted to cope with conflicting requirements of fire escape and security (see section 2.5.2). In any case fire evacuation from an enclosed area will need to be discussed and agreed with the appropriate authority.

Older people with dementia do not spend their time running riot but from time to time staff will need to cope with disturbed behaviour. In order to do so they need good contact with each other and good access to the resident. It is not uncommon for three people to be needed to manage a problem; one to distract, one to support and one to carry out whatever task needs doing. If the resident is in a wheelchair or seated in a special support chair a lot of space is needed. Spaces which are restricted by walls and furniture like toilets and bathrooms, corridors or dining rooms need careful consideration. There will be times when the residents will need to be attended by staff on each side. Cleaning people up after incontinence happens regularly. Staff will need to get someone who may be in a wheelchair out of a room into a bathroom or shower to wash and clean them. Clothing needs to be sluiced. It can be a daily frustration for staff if the doors are too narrow and swing the wrong way or if there is not enough room for a helper on each side of the toilet.

Any building for confused people must have things very firmly fixed to the walls. Normal fixings designed for domestic use are not appropriate. Anything which can be used as a handrail or grab rail will be used as such; this applies to towel rails or rings, washbasins or indeed anything within reach. Some fittings will be subjected to systematic 'abuse'. Sometimes the confused have a particular favoured activity which can be taking radiators off walls or dismantling door handles.

Guarding against accidental injury is of particular importance where demented people are accommodated as they will not be able to anticipate injury themselves or take remedial action if the injury occurs. Hot surfaces must be covered and falls from windows and stairs prevented. Handrail heights specified in the building regulations may not be high enough; some confused old people are very active and could climb over a metre high handrail at the top of a stair well. Doors and windows which minimize the risk of trapping

The people

A living room with glazed doors
giving easy access to a paved patio
and a secure but apparently
unrestricted garden.

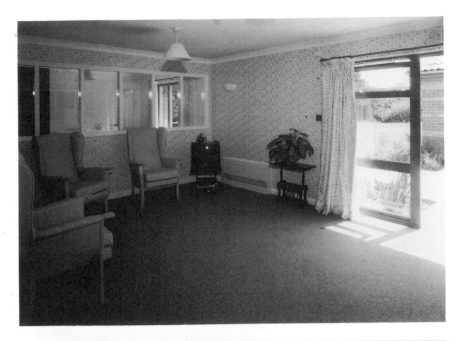

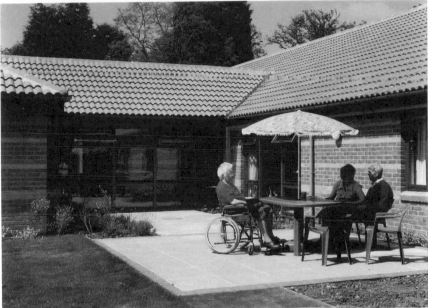

fingers should be specified. It is quite possible for a resident to close a window onto her own finger and leave it trapped, being unable to connect the pain with the action.

Behaviour to be accommodated

While nobody knows how to cure Alzheimer's disease there is a good knowledge of the kinds of behaviour which can be expected from a sufferer. Buildings for the demented should be designed to take into account the way people will behave, not frustrate them, and to make them comfortable in the endless present they inhabit.

Clarity of form and layout and good visibility are important. This is not particularly easy to achieve in a large residential building; there are many nursing and residential homes where the staff get disorientated from time to time, let alone the residents, particularly in bedroom corridors which can all appear identical with closed doors all round and not even a window to give a clue as to where you are. It is reasonable to assume that any residential building for more than 10 people will be confusing, not just to its dementia residents, and design techniques to counteract this are needed.

The route from bedrooms to day areas should be considered carefully. Dead ends and dog legs should be avoided; it should be obvious which way to go. Long corridors may be inevitable but they are not ideal. It is better if you can see the day areas from the bedrooms.

People like interesting places to sit. Interesting places are where things happen, so people will choose to sit in main entrances (even in a draught) watching service yards or at windows where something is going on outside. For someone who lives entirely in the present a constantly changing view of activity can be absorbing for long periods. Sitting areas can be planned to take advantage of the daily business generated by the home and the outside world.

Some people walk restlessly round the building in an apparently aimless way. A good range of safe wandering opportunities inside and out can be planned. They are of more value if they have some point to them, with distractions on route.

Reinforcement of reality

There is evidence that the confused and disorientated operate better when they know what is expected of them. Dining rooms should look like dining rooms, with tables laid, plates and crockery set, and bathrooms should look like bathrooms. This seems like stating the obvious, but often the requirements of communal living will produce spaces which cannot be immediately recognized. Dining may take place in sitting rooms; bathrooms may contain objects which look more like dentists chairs than baths. Special baths with integral lifting devices are excellent for bathing older people and avoid causing serious damage to the backs of the care assistants but can look alien and frightening to the confused person. While the bath may be essential it does not have to look as if it is in a clinic.

Older people may feel more at home in an old-fashioned environment. Most will come from homes which were furnished and decorated about thirty years ago. Radical modern furniture and decor will add to their confusion.

The bedroom is the only space which reflects the individual in a home, and it can be very personal. Everyone benefits from being surrounded by their own things: possessions can remind the confused of who they are and have therapeutic value. Bedrooms in residential homes are not large, and it is a design challenge to fit in all that is required (see section 2.2.2 Bed-sitting rooms.) Early decisions are required as to bedroom size and furniture. There are management advantages in having built-in furniture but many residents would prefer and benefit from the opportunity to bring in some of their own, perhaps a favourite chair or familiar dressing table. If residents are able to bring in their own furniture, storage will be needed for the spares, and there are issues which need to be discussed with registration and other authorities. Cherished arm chairs are rarely covered with flame-retarding fabrics and may be a bit tatty and at odds with the decor.

Confused residents often have difficulty finding their own bedroom. They all tend to look the same, especially in new homes. Ideally the living spaces should be next to and visible from the bedrooms, and individual bedrooms should be recognizable. Some homes provide residents with individual 'front' doors, which look like an external door with names, numbers, door bells and sometimes photographs on them. Colour or pattern can be used. Sometimes there is a problem in that residents can find the right room on the wrong floor, and it is helpful if areas of the building look distinctly different from each other.

The underlining of reality is helpful to the confused and every opportunity for highlighting use, function and time of day should be taken. Some homes are full of clocks, labels on doors and pictograms rather like the intake classes in primary schools on the principle that if the confused resident recognizes any of the objects this is a gain. Large institutions tend to produce bland interiors and a conscious effort is needed to counteract this effect.

The people

Dayrooms in a home based on family groups of 12 and 13. The scale and furnishings of the spaces are domestic and familiar looking

Top. Dining room and kitchenette

Bottom. Living room

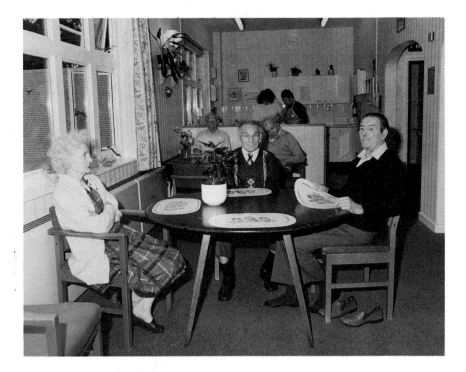

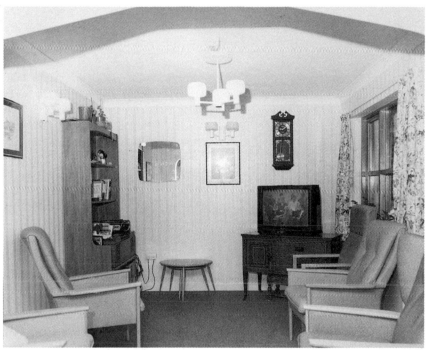

One of the symptoms of dementia is a reduced ability to learn new skills. It may be impossible for the confused person to learn how to use an unfamiliar artefact. A resident may never learn to operate a lever tap, or special door furniture designed for arthritic hands or other things outside their previous experience. There may be good reasons for specifying such items but it is worth making a critical assessment of their appropriateness. It helps if things look like an older person would expect them to look; this applies to doors and baths as much as to fittings and fixtures.

Colour, light and sound

People are attracted towards light places and it has been observed that confused people make for the light. Yet lighting, particularly daylighting design, is often poor in residential accommodation. The ideal organization of the building produces a layout with all spaces leading off the main day areas (entrance and administration wings, two or three bedroom wings, dining room links to kitchens), so day spaces tend to be surrounded by solid building with little opportunity for daylighting. Big roof spans produce deep plans. Add a few fire doors to separate compartments and it is only too easy to produce spaces entirely dependant on artificial light. Yet windows are clearly desirable in residential buildings. They provide light; they help people to orientate themselves in relation to the inside and outside of the building; they are interesting to look out of, particularly for those whose movement is restricted; they connect an introspective environment to the outside world, and they provide ventilation, essential in care homes.

The importance of good lighting quality means that light colours with high reflectance will be required, especially where rooms are deep and window areas small. Light bright and clear colours are indicated. The ability to distinguish between close hues, especially blue and green seems to deteriorate with age. This would suggest that subtle colour changes will not be so successful as contrasting colour. High lighting levels are required in all areas used by residents for reasons of safety and mobility as well as the need for people with failing sight to see and be seen. There is not much scope for gloomy atmospheric lighting design in a residential home.

The use of colour to differentiate parts of the building helps to orientate staff and residents and does not cost any extra. Identical bedroom corridors can be made to look very different from each other by use of colour and pattern. Contrasting colours on resident's doors are aids to recognition. Conversely doors can be disguised by painting them the same as the surrounding walls to discourage confused residents from using them if they lead to rooms which contain hazards.

Some people with dementia react badly to sudden changes in colour or pattern, and these should be avoided. Changes in floor colour or finish can be perceived as a step or hole in the ground which some will refuse to walk over. Highly patterned or realistic wallpaper can cause frustration; confused people may attempt to pick the 'flowers' off the wall and find it irritating when they fail. Bold stripes and even the lines which occur naturally in the building like handrails along a corridor can cause trouble. Problems have been reported with almost every kind of decoration: stripes, spots, flowers, bold and realistic patterns all have been criticized which leaves the designer in a quandary. The best option would appear to be fairly neutral designs in light clear colours.

Care homes can produce poor acoustic environments. Buildings which are open plan may have unacceptably high ambient sound levels. Noise can be coming from the television, other residents, nurse call bells, tables being laid, the kitchen, heating systems, water pipes as well as the care assistant who is trying to communicate with a resident. Dementia may cause a person to be quite unable to sort all this out. Good sound absorption and some sound reduction measures are needed.

Outside areas

Gardens in care homes are rarely fully exploited. Residents tend to sit inside even on the hottest days, yet potentially the outside has a lot to offer. There are opportunities for wandering paths which should be designed with incidents along the way, such as water splashes, or seats with views of the outside world. Valuable therapy can be conducted in vegetable gardens, greenhouses and sheds. It is good for someone who has been a life-time gardener to get the feel of soil in a plant pot.

Gardens need to be designed with the same care for safety as the rest of the building. Nearly all providers will want secure enclosures to prevent residents getting lost. Precautions against intruders may be necessary and grounds will need to be lit. Changes in level need guarding, and care must be taken in selection of planting material. Poisonous plants and plants with sharp thorns must be avoided. There is a list of poisonous and dangerous plants in Technical Supplement 3.

The people

Summary of key points

Location

- The building should be easily accessible for visiting; good access and transport links are desirable. Often former carers will have formed very strong bonds with people with dementia and may visit frequently. Visitors, particularly to specialist units, may have to come some distance. The best location from the point of view of residents is within or near to their own community on a public transport route so old friends as well as relatives can easily visit.
- The building should make the most of any activity taking place outside on the street. Sitting rooms and bedrooms and entrances should have a view of the outside world if at all possible, even if contrived; the service yard is more interesting to residents than the back garden.

Building layout

- Staff and residents need good visibility.
- Residents may be mobile and active. Good safe interesting wandering routes inside and outside are desirable.
- A high level of dependency is to be expected. Bathing, toilet and sluicing facilities should be of a high standard.
- A variety of spaces and activities should be accommodated. Residents will not spend all day sitting still.
- Some residents will be awake at night. Night staff need to be able to supervise them as well as sleeping residents.
- The building may need to respond to unconventional timetables; for instance, some residents may want food in the middle of the night.

Access and mobility

- Extra space is required for attendance on resident.
- Special furniture may be used for some residents. Chairs can be as big as 1 m × 2 m.
- Wide doors are preferred.
- Hold open devices will reduce the number of doors which have to be negotiated.
- Double swing doors may be required to toilets.

Interior detailed design

- Fittings need to be heavy duty and well fixed.
- Prevention measures against falling from windows and down stairs are required.
- Room functions should be obvious.

Environment

- Sound reduction and absorbency measures may be required.
- Good lighting is desirable.

Services

- Hot surfaces and pipes must be covered.
- Hot and cold taps should be marked or colour coded.

1.1.11 Ethnic minority groups

The tradition in most cultures, including those in Western Europe, is for families to take care of their ageing relatives at home. Most old people from different ethnic groups are cared for in this way. There are now a growing number of care homes specifically for the ethnic minorities. These homes are mainly developed by housing associations for a single race group of elderly people.

Designing for another culture needs sensitivity and is impossible without a good briefing team, with elders as well as younger people from the ethnic group represented. Older people from minority cultures are less likely to speak English, and have a stronger cultural identity than the generation which follows. People get old in similar ways, culture and race notwithstanding, and buildings for older people from ethnic minorities have similar requirements to any other care home. However, there are important other considerations which are specific to the culture and social framework which need to be addressed. What follows is a very brief summary of areas to be considered;

for further reading refer to the National Federation of Housing Associations (1993).

Location

Homes need to be near, or preferably within existing communities. The site chosen should be safe and secure. Areas where racial harassment causes problems should be avoided. The building must not become a target and should not draw attention to itself, but fit unobtrusively into its surroundings. Good lighting and boundaries are essential, with a clear definition of public and private areas. The public, street side should be well lit and easy to supervise visually day and night.

Building form

Most ethnic groups are from countries with warmer climates than Britain and traditional dwelling types have a relaxed relationship of inside to outside spaces. Courtyards, verandahs, porches and patios reflect lifestyles where much time is spent outdoors. Such forms, with the addition of suitable climate control can provide a basis for care home design. Briefing teams can provide information about traditional lifestyles.

Orientation and arrangement of the building in relation to the site may have significance for some groups. The relationship of buildings to Mecca is important to Moslems; toilets should not be aligned south east/north west. The foot of the bed should not point to Mecca. The orientation of the bed and its position in the bedroom is sacrosanct in many cultures and needs to be established early as it may be a restricting factor on the plan form.

Space requirements

Room layouts need to be discussed in detail at the planning stage to avoid expensive mistakes. There are cultural differences which affect most living spaces.

Dayrooms

- Large spaces may be required for group, social or religious meetings, or extended family gatherings. In some cultures there is segregation between the sexes and separated routes are needed to enable men to meet without encountering the women.
- Rooms may be used for specific rituals or religious practices.
- Links to outside areas may be important.

Washing and toilet areas

- Orientation may be important.
- Some religious ceremonies include ritual washing.
- Some cultures always bathe in running water, so showers may be appropriate. Floor finishes should be waterproof and sealed at skirtings.
- Bidets may be required.

Food preparation and dining

- Food storage requirements depend to some extent on diet. Large quantities of grains and dried goods may be consumed.
- Cooking methods may affect ventilation requirements.
- Some cultures handle different foods in separate areas.
- Religious ceremonies around ritual cooking and eating of food (for example the Passover) may require separate rooms and facilities.

Religious customs

- Family shrines or icons may be used. There are usually specific places where these should be sited.
- Prayer spaces may be needed.
- Regular ceremonies and rituals may have space or location requirements.
- Ritual washing may take place.

Circulation

- The building entrance often has significance. Space for shoes by the front door may be needed.
- The orientation of the stairs and their relationship to other spaces, particularly shrines may be sacrosanct.

Detailed design	• Signs should be in the right language particularly safety notices. • Some numbers and colours are avoided by different groups. • Certain built forms, for example arches may have particular meaning. • Security is of great importance. Ground floor windows, entrances and letter boxes may be targeted.
Outside areas	• Vegetable, herb and fruit growing areas are likely to be required. • Social areas out of doors are essential to many cultures. • Water gardens have symbolic meaning to some oriental cultures. • There are some planting taboos. Landscape and planting should be designed in full consultation with the briefing team.

1.2   Management structures

1.2.1 Owners and providers	The range of ownership patterns and management structures in care homes is large. This can be a problem for the designer as it is not always apparent who the client is. In many care homes management decisions are made by several people. When a new building is being commissioned it is important to formalize the briefing process. One person or a regular forum should make decisions. This can be hard to organize: often a large number of people are involved and if a key member of the team misses one meeting it can lead to abortive work. Some of the more common management structures are:
Private homes	At one end of the scale are small homes with owner/managers, sometimes living on site. Many homes are owned by doctors or nurses. Some owners run homes as family businesses which give a regular income and a capital asset to retire on. Others have plans for growth. Larger homes and groups of homes may be owned by individuals or companies. Operators who took advantage of the growth of the care homes market in the 1980s have been increasing their portfolios and may now manage groups of six to twelve homes. These are actively developing or acquiring new homes. The market leaders are publicly quoted companies with around fifty homes and include breweries and catering companies.
Voluntary homes	These include non-profit-making homes run by charities or housing associations. They vary widely in style and type of provision. Homes are managed by religious organizations, trades and professions, armed services charities and nationalist groups. Some have country-wide networks with national headquarters, others are small and local. Generally the homes are run by managers appointed by voluntary committees.
Local Authority homes and former Local Authority homes	These are former Old People's Homes, also known as Part Three homes. They are managed by the Social Services Departments of Local Authorities. Some Authorities continue to run their homes, others have transferred them to the independent sector. The homes that have been privatized are managed by non-profit-making trusts or charities, often formed by former staff of the Local Authority. The properties are transferred on a long lease, and the new organization has the task of raising capital to upgrade the existing stock. Most trusts have plans for expansion. The management structure is likely to have a social work rather than a medical bias.
NHS homes and homes under contract to NHS trusts	Health Authorities were traditionally providers of long-term care for mentally or physically frail older people. The role of hospitals is changing and now they are seen as providers of short-term acute care for the seriously ill. Hospitals still retain geriatric and psychogeriatric wards, but these are being phased out. NHS Trusts operate on a different basis from the former Health Authorities with their Estates Departments and are establishing new building

procurement routes. The major differences are that buildings are now expected to earn their keep so departments have to pay a capital charge for space they occupy, and private finance is being sought for new projects. Developments may be contracted out to the voluntary or private sector or run collaboratively between the NHS Trust and another organization, like a Housing Association. A typical arrangement is for the trust to select an operator on the basis of a tender to develop a scheme jointly. A site is made available on a long lease, the operator raises finance and the NHS guarantees to fill the beds at an agreed weekly fee. The NHS Trust retains an interest in the management of the home. Management structures are often complex, with people from different organizations represented, each with their own standing orders or quality standards. Projects are vulnerable to political pressures, last-minute budget cuts or policy changes on the one hand or, on the other, project financiers may require guarantees which the health trusts are unable to deliver.

The aims and objectives of the service provider need to be understood at the outset. Finance budgets and time frames and the relative priorities of capital growth or income will be discussed in detail at the early stages. Providers aiming to develop homes to sell on will favour low capital cost options over low running costs; others will take the opposite view. The type of residents to be catered for and proposed fee levels need to be identified. Long-term proposals for future expansion or alternative service provision need to be considered as well as current schemes.

While there are many different kinds of home, management structures of individual homes are similar. The diagram opposite shows typical management relationships.

Nursing homes differ from residential homes in that the manager and the person in charge at any time must be a doctor or a registered nurse.

1.2.2 Manager or matron

The manager or matron is responsible for the day-to-day running of the home. Some smaller homes are managed by their owners. Nursing homes must have a registered nurse on duty at all times, and many managers are of the nursing profession. The title matron, now an anachronism in the NHS is often used to give dignity to the position. Residential homes and voluntary homes are more likely to be managed by someone with a social work background and there are ideological differences between the two professions. The social workers argue that the nurses overprotect their clients, and that in the interests of individual freedom a certain degree of risk must be accepted. The two approaches to care have implications for the building design; while all clients will expect the building to be safe in the sense that obvious hazards are eliminated, there may be differing attitudes to supervision and containment of residents.

Few organizations are in a position to pay someone for a year to do nothing, so managers are often not appointed in time to be part of the briefing team for a new building, unless an existing home is being extended or developed. In the absence of the manager it is worth appointing a consultant with hands-on experience of running a home during the early stages.

The crucial nature of the manager's role is recognized in the legislation; managers have to be registered and approved by the registering authority as well as home owners. Managers are concerned with the day-to-day running of the home, setting standards and creating a good atmosphere, the appointment, training, management and motivation of staff, the quality of care given to the residents, relationships with residents, relatives, visitors, prospective clients and the general public. In building terms their requirements are a private office for administration, confidential records, interviews and meetings

The people

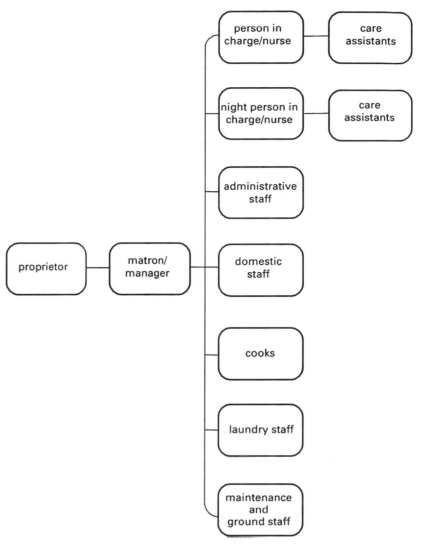

with staff. The location of the office should enable the manager to keep an overview of what is going on inside and outside the building.

1.2.3 Care staff

Care Assistants look after the residents. A few come to the job with nursing or social work qualifications, but the majority do not. Training is actively encouraged by registering authorities, and care assistants take NVQ courses while they are in post. The majority of care assistants are middle-aged women with school age or older children, working part time on shifts, although there are some men. Staff are often well motivated and do the work as much for the caring role as for the money. The workforce is more stable than would be expected given the low rates of pay which prevail.

Although pay rates are low, staff costs can take up to two thirds of the annual budget of a home. The ratio of staff to residents is laid down by the registering authority. It needs to be established at an early stage as it has a profound effect on the building layout. Homes organized in small family groups may need extra staff to supervise the residents adequately; each additional staff member will absorb most of the fee income from one resident.

Part-time shift workers often have family responsibilities and there is a strong preference for care assistants to work near their own homes. Care homes which are in residential areas find it relatively easy to recruit staff. The shift pattern means that some staff will be coming to work in the dark and it is important that they should feel safe. Special consideration is needed for the car parking areas and the route between them and the building. These spaces should be well lit and supervised.

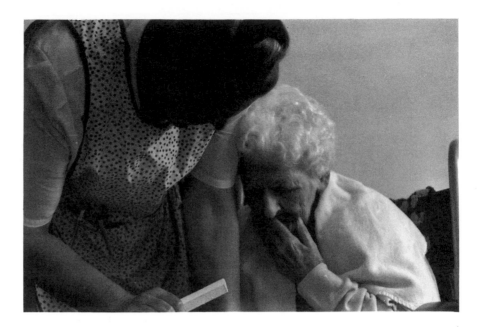

Staff accommodation must be in accordance with the Health and Safety at Work Act 1974 . The requirements are:

- a room for eating and rest separate from the residents;
- separate changing areas and toilets for male and female staff not shared with residents or with kitchen staff;
- cloak and locker provision.

Locker and cloak space sometimes causes a problem. Both sets of shift workers will be present during staff changeovers which can mean a lot of coats and handbags.

Staff accommodation rarely gets the attention that other parts of the building command at the briefing stage, but there are some important issues to be resolved. Some providers take the view that staff should essentially spend their time with the residents and staff accommodation should be no more than adequate. They feel that a comfortable staff room will mean extended breaks to the detriment of resident care. Residents can feel excluded in homes where the relationships between staff are particularly good; the home can seem to be run more for the benefit of the staff than the residents. A counter argument is that a happy staff means a happy home: 'look after the staff and they will look after the resident' is written into the Domus policy document (HMSO, 1992).

Staff areas are usually provided with tea-making facilities and a sink. The smoking issue should be addressed at the briefing stage; care home staff, like nurses are dedicated smokers. Some homes have a non-smoking policy. These can be recognized by the small groups of desperate residents and staff having a cigarette outside one of the fire escape doors. Others have smoking lounges with good extract fans where residents and staff may smoke.

Care homes are sometimes criticized for using unqualified and untrained staff. Senior staff who have the qualifications and training spend the bulk of their time in administration, so the residents do not directly gain from their experience. Quality standards are being encouraged and improved staff training will follow. Staff rooms may be required to double as training rooms.

Staff care for residents physically and socially and do some domestic and cleaning tasks. They need good access to the residents, and to have good visual supervision, though it is important that these requirements do not impinge on the residents' need for a sense of privacy.

Care homes have a 24-hour day with waking staff doing night shifts. The buildings should feel safe at night. Systems and controls need to be user friendly and reliable. Night-time emergencies should be confined to problems with the residents, not the building.

The health hazards associated with the job are back injuries, infections and sometimes attacks by the residents. Back injuries are caused by lifting with a bent back, and occur most frequently bathing residents or picking them up after a fall. Some residents can be very heavy and at times uncooperative. A single female should not lift a weight over five stone (32 kg), and two women together should not attempt to lift over eight stone (51 kg). Heavier weights need hoists or lifting aids. Written safety policy documents with risk assessment should be adopted by managers, and staff trained in safe lifting techniques. If hoists are to be used they will need to be stored when not in use. For the dimensions of commonly used hoists and special baths see section 2.2.3.

Prevention of cross-infection is a priority for care homes whose residents are particularly vulnerable to outbreaks of food poisoning. Hand washing and drying facilities, separate from the residents are required, particularly where staff may handle soiled linen or residents. Care staff should keep out of the kitchens, and separate toilets and washing facilities are needed for kitchen staff.

1.2.4 Domestic staff

Some domestic duties are undertaken by the care assistants and other ancillary staff are employed to do the cooking, cleaning, laundry, administration and routine building and ground maintenance. Alternatively some of these tasks may be performed by outside contractors. Domestic staff have an important role in relation to the residents.

Checklist of staff requirements:

Location
- good access to local housing areas;

Building layout
- staff room, separate exclusive toilets, cloaks and shower area for males and females to be provided; good visibility for unobtrusive supervision;
- space for handling and assisting residents; space for a care assistant on each side of resident in toilets, bathroom, corridors; doors need to be wide enough;
- lifting aids and special baths to be specified in initial stages; storage space for equipment to be assessed;

Services
- control systems to be designed for non-technical operators;

Site layout
- good security and site lighting required for late shift workers.

1.3 Regulators

The registration procedure is described in section 3.1.1. This section deals with the personnel involved.

1.3.1 Inspectors and Registration Officers

Nursing homes

Nursing homes are inspected and registered by the District Health Authorities. The Inspection Officers appointed by the Authorities register new or altered homes, homes which change ownership or management, and carry out at least two inspections of homes per year. Inspection Officers may have a medical or health care background. They are usually supported by technical staff who advise on building and services, and draw on the resources of the Authority for other advice. The Inspectors also investigate complaints.

The inspectorate also has an educational function. Training and advice to home owners and managers is offered, and sometimes courses are run.

Inspectors may also be involved in briefing, particularly for new NHS developments.

Residential homes	Residential homes are inspected by the Local Authority. Inspection Officers operate in a similar way to their counterparts in the Health Authorities. They are likely to have a social work background. Where homes are dual registered the Authorities work together to ensure both sets of guidelines are met.
Lay Assessors	Both Health Authorities and Local Authorities are encouraged to appoint Lay Assessors of care homes. These are members of the public who are independent of the Registering Authorities. They work with the inspection units, attending inspections of homes and contribute to the formal report. They are appointed to bring a non-professional perspective to the assessment of homes.

1.3.2 Other officials

Fire Officer	In order to obtain registration the Fire Officer has to give written confirmation that the fire precautions are in accordance with the Building Regulations and other requirements. Once the home is occupied the Fire Officer will inspect it annually, make recommendation for any work that is required and state a date by which essential work must be done.
Environmental Health Officer	Food safety and hygiene arrangements must be approved in writing by the Environmental Health Officer before a home can be registered. Their remit covers food storage preparation and distribution, kitchen staff hygiene, laundry and collection and storage of soiled linen and clothing, washing and toilet facilities for staff, residents and visitors.
Planning Officer	The Planning Officer is required to confirm that a development or extension has Planning Approval, and that all the conditions on the Approval have been met.
Building Control Officer	Formal confirmation is required from the Building Control Officer that the building or any extension or alteration complies with the Building Regulations.
Community Pharmacist	The Community Pharmacist advises on the correct storage and administration of drugs, including security measures required.

1.4 The outside world

1.4.1 Personal visitors

Some residents are visited regularly, daily or weekly, others rarely or never. Where there is a regular visitor it is likely to be one person, perhaps a daughter or son who lives nearby. Other family members tend to visit much less frequently. Visitors tend to be in the 60–70 age group, and some residents will be visited by friends of their own age. Children do visit homes but not very frequently, although a home in East Anglia has a swimming pool which tends to increase child participation in and enthusiasm for visiting. Volunteers are sometimes asked to visit people who have no other outside contacts.

The complaint of visitors and relatives is that they feel excluded. Sometimes relatives have carried the load of caring for someone before residential care was taken up. The move can leave the relatives bereft, and many feel guilty. They no longer seem to have a purpose, they see others carrying out all the caring tasks, and they can even be excluded from health decisions made by doctors and staff on behalf of their relatives.

Successful caring regimes are those where the elderly retain as much autonomy and control over their lives as possible. Individuals need their own private territory, relationships and possessions. Family relationships are part of what defines the individual. They are fragile and need to be handled with care. An institution with its own compelling agenda of timetables and staff efficiency can shatter and spoil relationships which become formal and stilted. Some homes recognize this and work in partnership with relatives and friends. Needs of visitors are recognized and given due importance; they should be written into the building brief and management objectives. This is an area which has been neglected; homes have been designed with other priorities. The presence of relatives' representatives and other non-professionals on Local and Health Authority inspection teams and new quality assurance initiatives may do something to shift the emphasis.

What visitors may require includes:

Location

- Good access. Not all visitors have cars. Ideally homes should be located in residential areas with good transport links. This is essential for peer group visits.

Building layout

- Easy routes for residents to be taken out in their visitor's cars. Car parks or disabled parking bays should be near the main entrance with handrails.
- Privacy. Visitors should be able to see their relatives in a private place. Small lounges may be appropriate. The resident's own room is best, provided there is enough space.
- Spaces where relaxed social exchanges can take place. It is easy to talk over a drink, a meal, a game of cards or snooker or on a walk round a garden. It is almost impossible in a large quiet room surrounded by twenty inquisitive strangers.
- Privacy to speak to the manager or staff. Confidential issues can be discussed concerning financial arrangements and health, or the relatives may want to make a complaint. It is hard to do this effectively in a public lounge surrounded by people.
- Space to grieve. Many old people will die while in a home. Their relatives may wish to be with them, or are likely to visit soon after a death.
- Courtesy. Minor discomforts can make people feel unwelcome and can make the visit something to be endured rather than enjoyed. Careful design and management regimes can go a long way to overcome this. Visitors should be able to get a cup of tea or a meal without feeling they have disrupted the homes' routine.
- Contact with other relatives. Visiting relatives appreciate a forum where they can communicate. This can be a simple bulletin board or a space for occasional meetings.
- Reception and entrance areas are not always well handled. Sometimes visitors have to run the gauntlet of curious old people sitting round the door avid for entertainment. While this is good for the residents it can be daunting for visitors. Gaining access to the building can be a problem. Some homes have receptionists sitting near the front door; in others it is not uncommon to ring the bell and have the door opened by a passing care assistant who immediately disappears. In homes with entryphones sometimes nobody comes to the door at all.

1.4.2 Community visitors

- Registration Authorities encourage homes to make good links with the community. Visitors will be encouraged, to give entertainments or conduct religious services or carol singing. Community visitors share the same needs as relatives for good reception and sometimes privacy. There is also a need for a social space for the big occasions. This can be a problem if the home is organized in family groups.

1.4.3 Working visitors

Some professional visitors have specific requirements:

Building layout

- Ministers of religion may require a space for conducting a service for all the residents. The largest lounges are used. Space is needed for all residents,

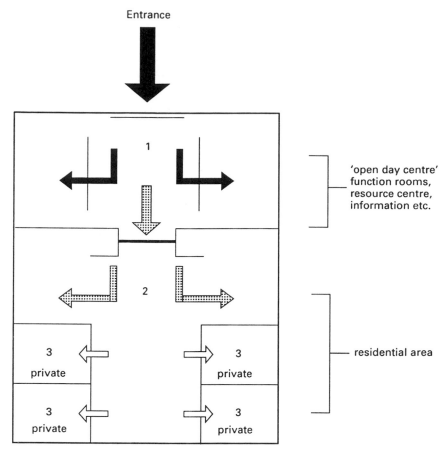

Entrance

'open day centre' function rooms, resource centre, information etc.

residential area

1   Open centre/semi-public
A fairly 'Open door' through which anyone in the community can pass, who has a reason for doing so, e.g. go for day care, attend a coffee morning or ask for information.

2   Residential areas
Closed to members of general public and only open to people who have a reason to go through – residents, visitors, staff etc.

3   Private rooms
The residents' private space, the threshold of which no one passes, including staff, without seeking and gaining permission. Residents have their own key.

Arthur Neal House, an EPICS (Elderly People's Integrated Care System) centre. A former Local Authority Part Three home which has been successfully adapted using the principles of progressive privacy to form a day centre for older people offering integrated services in the public part of the home while continuing to provide residential care in the private areas

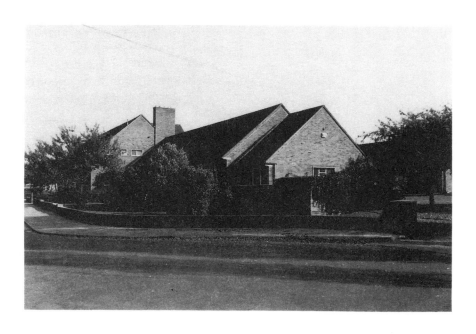

allowing for some to be in wheelchairs. Care staff will be in attendance. The group will focus on the minister. Good visibility and acoustic design is needed.

- Health professionals such as doctors and community nurses, physiotherapists, occupational therapists and chiropodists and sometimes dentists and optometrists will visit. Individuals are usually seen in their own rooms. Sometimes there is a treatment room and the individual professions may need space allocated although they are likely to bring their own kit with them. NHS homes will have more specific requirements, and the various professionals should be on the briefing team. If they do not turn up they need to be pursued. It is sometimes difficult to fit a full chiropody suite into a building just before the tenders go out.
- A hairdresser will probably visit regularly and will require a hairdressing sink with a mirror and shelf space. This can be located in a bathroom, a corner of a lounge, a semi-screened area or a dedicated room. The weekly hairdo is something of a treat, and the space should have the atmosphere of a salon.

Services

- Services and lifts installations have to be regularly inspected and tested, and building maintenance and upgrading is an ongoing process. This can make homes very public places. It is important that visiting operatives understand the need to respect individual privacy, to knock before entering rooms and to make sure that the residents' dignity is maintained. Contracts should have clauses written in which make this clear.

1.4.4 Day-care visitors

Care homes are obvious places for providing day-care facilities and there are good reasons for so doing. The home can benefit from stronger links with the community; there is a normalizing influence. People who become resident are more comfortable about moving in if they are already familiar with the home. The building is staffed and equipped to provide for the needs of older people. The danger is that the day-care provision can be at the expense of the resident population. There are territorial conflicts, and the residents can feel threatened and invaded in what is, in fact, their only home.

The users of day care are older people living near the home who are assessed as needing additional support without full residential care. The kind of support provided needs to be accurately defined, and tailored to the building provision. The needs may be social contact, meals provision, health care and hygiene. The day-care provision on site can be extended to a peripatetic service.

Building brief

The concept of progressive privacy has been developed by Richard Hollingbery whilst Director of the Helen Hamlyn Foundation, a charitable trust which specializes in developing holistic models of care for frail older people. Permanent residents can feel invaded by day-care visitors encroaching on their territory. The principle of progressive privacy should prevent this problem. The following is an extract reproduced with permission from design guidelines produced by the Foundation (Hollingbery, 1993).

Progressive privacy

There are three types of space:

1 Open centre/semi-public: a fairly 'open door' through which anyone in the community can pass, who has a reason for doing so, e.g. for day care, attend a coffee morning or ask for information.
2 Residential areas: closed to members of the general public, and only open to people who have a reason to go through, e.g. residents, visitors, staff.
3 Private rooms: the resident's private space – the threshold of which no one passes, including staff – without seeking and gaining permission. Residents have their own keys.

Each area is defined by its own door/ entrance.

Progressive privacy facilitates the integration of a number of uses within the same building, i.e. no separate entrances for different people. It allows access to all parts of the building without disturbing other activities.

It familiarizes (older) people with the building, so that they can come to the same place for different purposes, i.e. it eases the transition between different types of care.

It allows residents to 'go out', e.g. to the activity areas or restaurant without leaving the building. It promotes choice as to where and with whom the residents spend their time.

The public spaces will include rooms for treatment, such as chiropody, assisted bathing facilities, toilets and services like hairdressing. Dining areas must have sufficient space for visitors without interfering with the residents who will be unwilling to vacate their usual places. Catering and kitchen arrangements need to be very flexible. It is impossible to predict day-care numbers with any accuracy. Social areas must be separate from and in addition to the resident's private day areas. These can be used for group activities like bingo, card schools, religious services, concerts and parties. Access and parking needs to be good and the entrance generous. The plan of the building should make it clear to strangers which are the public areas and which are not.

1.4.5   Respite care

Respite care visitors may stay for a few days or weeks. They are likely to be integrated into the life of the home. Their needs are similar to the other residents; respite care may precede an eventual move into the home.

2 Building design guide

2.1 Anthropometrics

Anthropometric data for older people

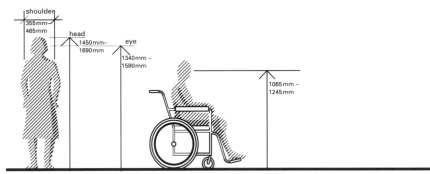

physical dimensions   eye level wheelchair

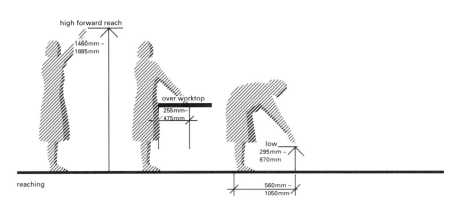

reaching

Wheelchair dimensions (attendant-
and self-propelled)

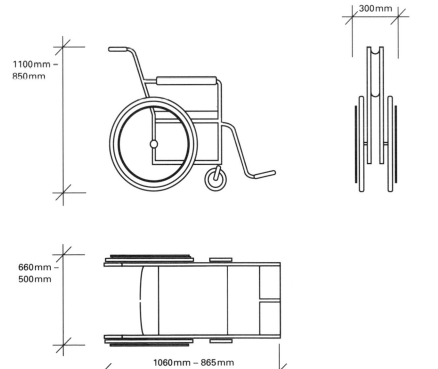

2.2 Activity and space requirements

2.2.1 Circulation

(a) Circulation spaces

User requirements

Residents

- Short travel routes preferred.
- View of destination desirable.
- Space for wheelchairs to pass each other.
- Handrail to both sides, continuous if possible.
- No level changes.
- Circulation spaces differentiated from each other to avoid confusion.
- Windows in circulation routes aid orientation.
- Absence of obstacles along the way.
- Transition zone from public space to private rooms.
- Private functions to be protected from public view.
- Minimum corridor width may be specified.

Care staff

- Good visual supervision.
- Space to assist residents while passing trolleys, wheelchairs etc.
- Monitoring of movement through fire escape doors (dementia units).

Interior

Finishes

- Impervious carpet.
- Domestic decorations.
- Protection against wheelchair and trolley damage.

Fittings

- Handrails.
- Fire extinguishers.

Furniture

- Preferably no unfixed furniture because of fire risk.

Services

Heating

- Recommended temperature 21°C.
- Low temperature heat emitters, maximum surface temperature 43°C.
- Handrails to avoid heaters.

Electrics

- Power points for cleaning.

Systems

- Nurse call with reset and assistance request.
- Room call indicator lights.
- Room presence indicator lights.
- Smoke detector indicator lights in roof space, lift shaft and other remote spaces.
- Additional smoke detection may be required if automatic door hold open devices installed.
- Fire alarm call points at exits.
- Exit door opening monitors.

Environment

Lighting

- CIBSE interior lighting code recommended level for corridors: 20–100 lux, low level late night lighting with override facility (where residents are likely to be disturbed at night 100 lux is appropriate day and night).
- CIBSE interior lighting code recommended level for stairs: 100 lux, higher in hazardous areas (there should be a contrast between treads and risers; light coloured contrasting nosings improve safety.)
- No glare or shiny reflective surfaces (CIBSE code limiting glare index 19).
- End destinations and corners or transition zones highlighted.
- Emergency lighting.
- Illuminated exit signs.

Acoustics

- Sound reduction for impact sound between floors or privacy between rooms and corridors.

Building elements

Windows

- Views out of circulation spaces to orientate building users.
- Opening restrictors for first floor windows and above.
- Security for ground floor windows.
- Curtains or blinds.

Doors

- 1000 mm wide doors preferred for wheelchair access, required by some authorities; minimum 900 mm.

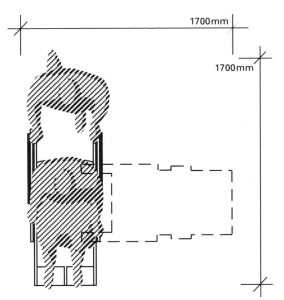

1700mm

1700mm

wheelchair turning circle (assisted)

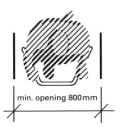

min. opening 800mm

person using walking aid

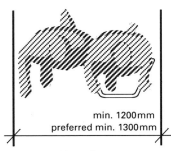

min. 1200mm
preferred min. 1300mm

walking with assistant

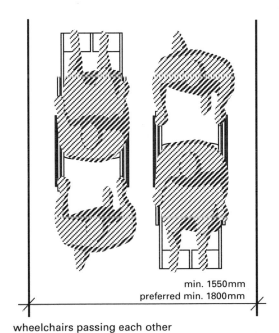

min. 1550mm
preferred min. 1800mm

wheelchairs passing each other

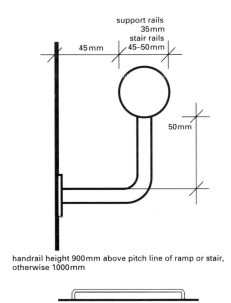

support rails
35mm
stair rails
45–50mm

45mm

50mm

handrail height 900mm above pitch line of ramp or stair,
otherwise 1000mm

handrail to be returned into wall at the ends to avoid
catching clothing or handbags

Top and bottom left, and top right. Circulation dimensions

Bottom right. Handrail dimensions

- Unrestricted openings preferred if fire precautions and privacy requirements permit.
- Vision panels in doors which have to be closed.

Ironmongery
- Self-closers may be required, but are powerful; automatic hold open devices linked to the fire alarm preferred but expensive.
- Conflicting requirements of fire escape, security and containment of confused residents to be resolved for external doors.
- Lever handles.
- Door and architrave protection reduces trolley and wheelchair damage.

(b) Reception and entrance areas

Location

- Near main entrance.
- Obvious to visiting strangers.
- Easy access to car, taxi and ambulance parking.
- Visitors toilets and cloaks space nearby.
- Near space for private interviews and meetings.
- Access to public telephone.

User requirements

Residents

- Draught-proof sitting areas overlooking the entrance.

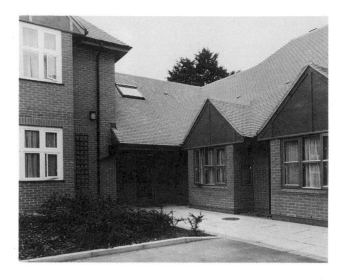

Rooms overlooking the entrance give residents a chance to watch some activity

Administrative staff

- Reception and discrete screening of visitors.

Visitors

- Reception and welcome.
- Private interviews with manager or staff.

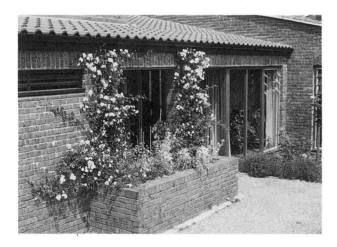

Entrance under recessed porch. Liscombe House, PRP Architects, 1976–1977

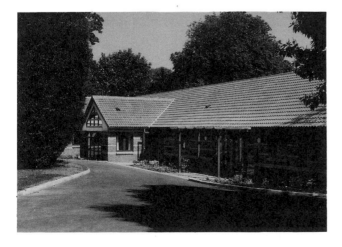

A wheelchair-friendly entrance with a drop-off point for vehicles

Emergency services

- Fire alarm indicator panel and plan of building by front door.

Interior

Finishes

- Impervious carpet.
- Entrance matting of sufficient depth to clean wheelchair wheels (1.9 m minimum).

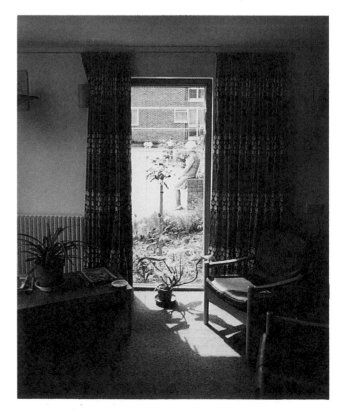

Reception area. Liscombe House, PRP Architects, 1976–1977

- Good standard of decoration (visitors get first impression of home here).

Fittings
- Reception desk or hatch.
- Notice board.
- Handrails.
- Fire extinguishers.
- Fixed seating in entrance.
- Mail box.

Furniture
- Easy chairs.
- Coffee table.

Services
Heating
- Recommended temperature 23°C.
- Low temperature heat emitters, maximum surface temperature 43°C.

Electrics
- Power points for cleaning.

Systems
- Fire alarm panel and zoned building plan in entrance.
- Smoke detectors.
- Fire alarm call point at entrance.
- Entryphone or other access monitoring system.
- Door bell linked to nurse call system.
- Door opening alarm linked to nurse call system.
- Security monitor.

Environment
Lighting
- CIBSE interior lighting code recommended levels: enquiry desks 500 lux, limiting glare index 19 (could be localized lighting); main entrance 200 lux, limiting glare index 19.
- Emergency lighting.
- Illuminated exit sign.

Acoustics
- Sound proofing to private interview space.

Building elements
Windows
- Additional security for windows.
- Curtains or blinds.

Doors
- Entrance door wide enough for frequent wheelchair use; double doors or automatic opening doors a possibility.
- Flush threshold.
- Large glazed panels are inappropriate; vision panels or glazing bars needed.

Ironmongery
- Secure locking compatible with fire escape.
- If door closers installed, they should not prevent old people from opening doors.
- Door and architrave protection to prevent wheelchair and trolley damage.
- Draught-proof letter plate.
- Ironmongery to deter confused residents from opening entrance door (e.g. additional lever handle at high level or electric release controllable by staff or visitors with automatic release when the fire alarm sounds); all anti-wandering devices to be discussed with and approved by the Fire Prevention Officer.

(c) Lifts and lift machine rooms
Location
- Lifts should be convenient for main circulation routes, day rooms, bed-sitting rooms and main entrance. A central location is preferred.
- Check manufacturer's recommendations on location of lift machine room in relation to lift.
- Check manufacturer's recommendation for minimum safe head room for maintenance staff above top of lift.
- Size of lift pit and head room may restrict available lift positions.
- Check ventilation requirements for machine room.

User requirements
Residents
- User-friendly lift, 8-person minimum size.
- Smooth ride.
- Wheelchair access.

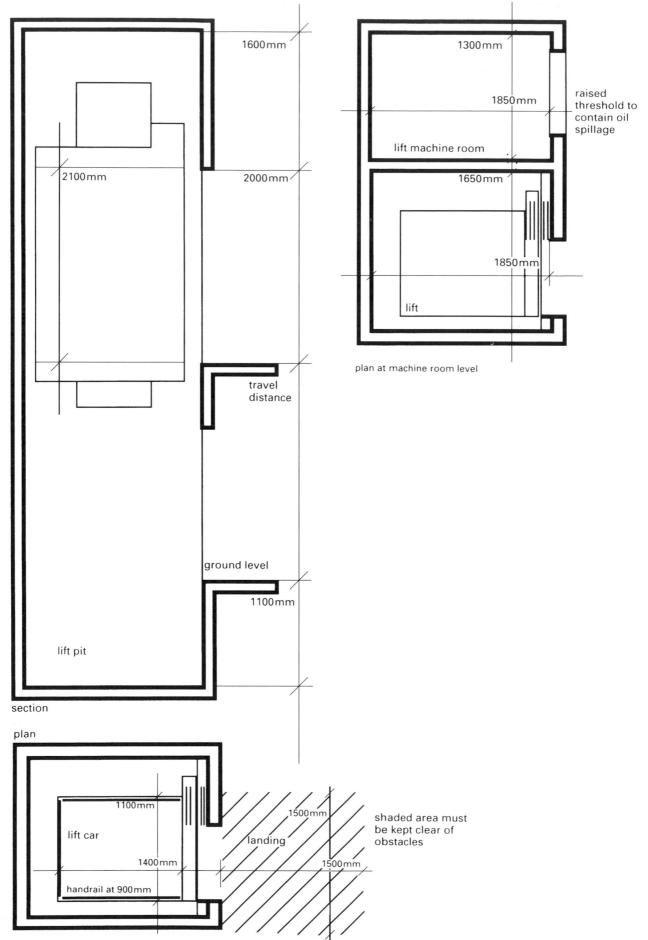

1600mm

2100mm

2000mm

travel
distance

ground level

1100mm

lift pit

section

plan

1100mm

lift car

1400mm

handrail at 900mm

landing

1500mm

1500mm

shaded area must
be kept clear of
obstacles

1300mm

1850mm

lift machine room

raised
threshold to
contain oil
spillage

1650mm

1850mm

lift

plan at machine room level

Eight-person hydraulic lift Minimum shaft and machine room dimensions. The machine room can be located on any floor, preferably adjacent to the lift shaft

- Accurate levelling at floor.
- High lighting level without glare.
- Handrail in lift.
- Control panel accessible to wheelchair passengers (maximum height 1.2 m).
- Controls suitable for people with poor eyesight.
- Emergency call system.
- Emergency hand-lowering.
- Extended door-opening time control.
- Reliability.

Interior
Finishes
- Non-slip floor.
- Light and bright interior.

Fittings
- Handrail.

Services
Electrics
- Design and installation to comply with BS 5655.
- 3-phase supply required.

Systems
- Smoke or heat detection at top of lift shaft with visual indicators on floor below.
- Smoke and or heat detectors in lift machine room with visual indicators outside room.
- Fire alarm.

Environment
Lighting
- CIBSE interior lighting code recommended level 100 lux.
- BS 5655 (38) Part 1 specifies minimum illumination of 50 lux on car floor.

Acoustics
- Sound buffers or sound reduction for noisy lift machine rooms.

Building elements
Walls
- Lift shaft fire protection to roof level.

- Check manufacturer's recommendations for structural support (some lifts have independent steel structures).
- Tanking to below-ground lift pits.

Doors
- 800 mm clear wide door to lift for minimum wheelchair provision (830 mm preferred).
- Threshold for oil spillage containment required for hydraulic lift machine room.

Ironmongery
- Lockable door to machine room.

2.2.2 Residents' living areas
(a) Bed-sitting rooms, apartments
Location
- Route between bed-sitting rooms and dayrooms to be short and obstacle free (for people to see their destination).
- Bedroom windows with interesting view.
- Small lounges nearby for the use of residents who wake at night (night staff need to monitor activity or disturbance in bed-sitting rooms).

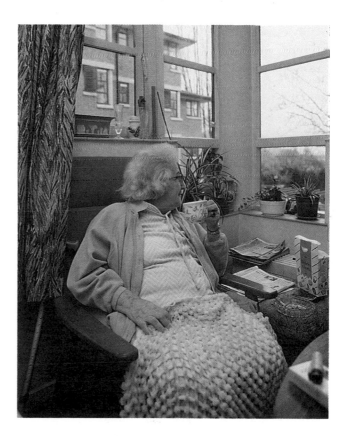

Bed-sitting room. St Mark's Road, Kensington, PRP Architects, 1989

- En-suite with toilet and washing or shower facility where possible.

User requirements
Residents
- Room to reflect owner's personality.
- Room door to convey personal territory is entered here.
- Rooms possibly furnished with residents' possessions.
- Bed-sitting rooms sized to entertain visitors.
- Interesting view.
- Security for personal possessions.
- Small number of double rooms for couples or siblings (adjacent rooms with interconnecting doors can be furnished as a flatlet for two people).
- Minimum space standards mandatory.

Care staff
- Space for nursing and bed making on each side of the bed.
- Separate staff facilities for handwashing.
- Residents to be monitored at night without disturbance or intrusion of their privacy.

Interior
Finishes
- Impervious carpet.
- Domestic decorations.

Fittings
- Wash hand basin or vanity unit if not provided in en-suite bathroom.
- Lever or cross top taps.
- Waste plug to be omitted if there is a risk of taps being left on.
- Thermostatic mixer controls.
- Grab rail.
- Towel rail (will be used as grab rail).
- Soap dish.
- Soap dispenser.
- Hand dryer or towel dispenser and bin.
- Toothbrush holder.
- Mirror.
- Shaving point and mirror light with pull cord.
- Wall light.
- Picture rail or alternative method of fixing pictures.

Furniture
- Bed (divan or hospital type) – preferred height 480 mm for wheelchair and semi-ambulant users, 450 mm for mobile users, 680 mm for nursing access.
- Cot sides (for use where there is risk of falling out of bed).
- Armchairs.
- Commode.
- Wardrobe (built-in, free-standing or resident's own).
- Chest of drawers (built-in, free-standing or resident's own).
- Table.
- Locker.
- Television.
- Shelves for ornaments, photographs etc.

Services
Heating
- Recommended temperature 23°C.
- Low temperature heat emitters, maximum surface temperature 43°C.

Hot and cold water
- Hot water delivered at a nominal maximum of 43°C within the band 41–45°C.
- Thermostatic mixers with fail safe devices within 2 m of each hot water outlet.
- Covered hot pipes.
- Cold water (potable).
- Stop valves if required.

Electrics
- Power points for cleaning, bedhead, tv etc.

Systems
- Nurse call with reset and assistance request.
- Smoke detector.
- Telephone point.
- TV aerial point and video channel.
- Non-intrusive methods for night-time monitoring (e.g. infrared movement sensors or pressure pads adjacent to bed).

Environment
Lighting
- Lighting at bedhead and general lighting.

- CIBSE interior lighting code recommended level 100 lux.
- Dimmer switch if required.
- Low level night lighting for staff to check residents if required.

Acoustics

- Agreed sound reduction index between rooms (at 40 dB loud speech can be heard but not distinguished; at 45 dB loud speech can be heard faintly but not distinguished; at 50 dB shouting can only be heard with difficulty).

Ventilation

- Fast ventilation required to air room.

Building elements
Windows

- Unobstructed view from bed and armchair.
- No glazing bars at eye level.
- Opening restrictors for first floor windows and above.
- Windows lockable in the open vent position to prevent injury.
- Security for ground floor windows.
- Curtain.

Doors

- 1000 mm wide doors preferred for wheelchair access, and required by some authorities, minimum width 900 mm.
- Identification of individual front doors with photographs, nameplates or colour.

Ironmongery

- Self closers may be required, but are too powerful; automatic hold open devices linked to the fire alarm preferred but expensive.
- Lever handles.
- Locks with emergency lock releases.

(b) Guest bedrooms
Location

- En-suite bathroom with toilet and washing or shower facility, or within reach of bathroom and toilet.

User requirements
Guests

- Clothes hanging space.

Interior
Finishes

- Carpet.
- Domestic decorations.

Fittings

- Wash hand basin or vanity unit if not provided in en-suite bathroom.
- Lever or cross top taps.
- Thermostatic mixer controls.
- Towel rail.
- Soap dish.
- Toothbrush holder.
- Mirror.

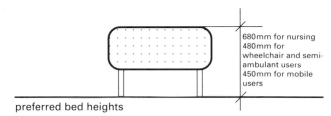

680mm for nursing
480mm for wheelchair and semi-ambulant users
450mm for mobile users

preferred bed heights

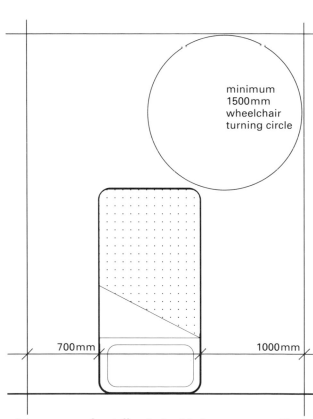

minimum 1500mm wheelchair turning circle

700mm   1000mm

minimum space for staff and wheelchair access around bed

Access around bed

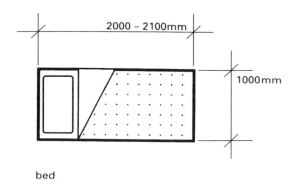

2000 – 2100mm

1000mm

bed

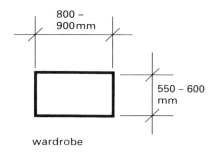

800 – 900mm

550 – 600 mm

wardrobe

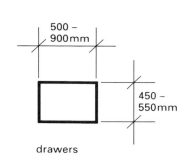

500 – 900mm

450 – 550mm

drawers

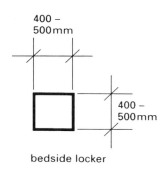

400 – 500mm

400 – 500mm

bedside locker

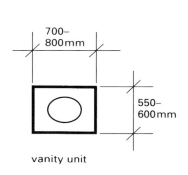

700 – 800mm

550 – 600mm

vanity unit

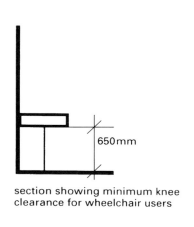

650mm

section showing minimum knee clearance for wheelchair users

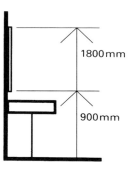

1800mm

900mm

top and bottom of mirror suitable for ambulant and wheelchair users

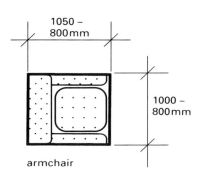

1050 – 800mm

1000 – 800mm

armchair

Bedroom furniture with range of furniture sizes. It is best to establish exact dimensions early when minimum room areas are adopted. Allow more space if residents are to use their own furniture

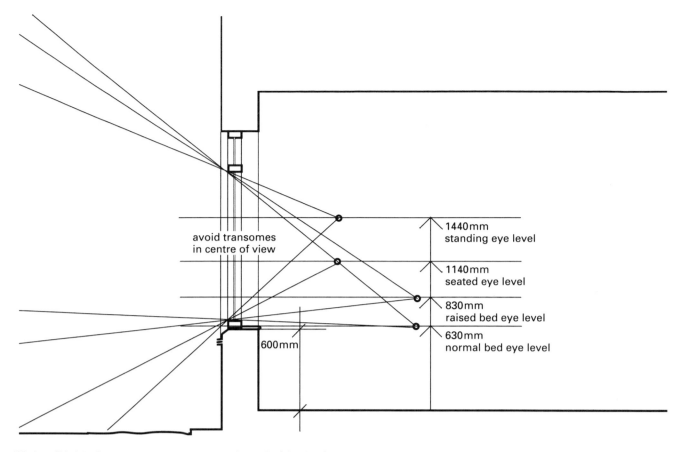

avoid transomes
in centre of view

1440mm
standing eye level

1140mm
seated eye level

830mm
raised bed eye level

630mm
normal bed eye level

600mm

Window cill height. Even cills as low as 600 mm restrict much of the view for someone in bed

- Shaving point and mirror light with pull cord.
- Wall light.

Furniture
- Bed.
- Armchair.
- Wardrobe.
- Chest of drawers.
- Bedside table.
- Locker.

Services
Heating
- Recommended temperature 23°C.
- Low temperature heat emitters, maximum surface temperature 43°C.

Hot and cold water
- Hot water delivered at a nominal maximum of 43°C within the band 41–45°C.
- Thermostatic mixers with fail safe devices within 2 m of each hot water outlet.
- Hot pipes covered.

- Cold water (potable).
- Stop valves if required.

Electrics
- Power point for cleaning, bedhead.

Systems
- Smoke detector.

Environment
Lighting
- Lighting at bedhead and general lighting.
- CIBSE interior lighting code recommended level 100 lux.

Acoustics
- Agreed sound reduction index between rooms (at 40 dB loud speech can be heard but not distinguished; at 45 dB loud speech can be heard faintly but not distinguished; at 50 dB shouting can only be heard with difficulty).

Building elements
Window

- Opening restrictors for first floor windows and above.
- Security for ground floor windows.
- Curtain.

Doors

- 1000 mm wide doors preferred for wheelchair access, and required by some authorities, minimum width 900 mm.

Ironmongery

- Self closers if required.
- Lever handles.
- Lock with emergency release.

(c) Close care flats
Location

- Within reasonable walking distance of dayrooms (residents in close care flats are not so dependant on communal facilities).
- Windows with interesting view.
- En-suite bathroom with toilet and washing or shower facility.

User requirements
Residents

- Flat to reflect owner's personality.
- Door to convey personal territory is entered here.
- Rooms possibly furnished with residents' possessions.
- Flats sized to entertain visitors.
- Interesting view.
- Security for personal possessions.
- Space for two beds if required for couples or siblings.
- Kitchenette for preparation of light meals or drinks (main meals are likely to be taken in the main dining room).

Care staff

- Space for nursing and bed making on each side of bed.
- Separate staff facilities.

Interior
Finishes

- Impervious carpet.
- Non-slip vinyl or PVC to en-suite toilet and kitchenette.
- Domestic decorations.

Fittings

- Wash hand basin or vanity unit.
- Lever or cross top taps.
- Thermostatic mixer controls.
- Grab rail.
- Towel rail (will be used as grab rail).
- Soap dish.
- Soap dispenser.
- Hand dryer or towel dispenser and bin.
- Toothbrush holder.
- Mirror.
- Shaving point and mirror light with pull cord.
- Wall light.
- Sink unit.
- Refrigerator.
- Small cooker, microwave oven or hob.

Furniture

- Bed (divan or hospital type) – preferred height 480 mm for wheelchair and semi-ambulant users, 450 mm for mobile users, 680 mm for nursing access.
- Wardrobe (built-in, free-standing or resident's own).
- Chest of drawers (built-in, free-standing or resident's own).
- Bedside table.
- Locker.
- Armchairs.
- Television.
- Small dining table.
- Shelving.
- Sideboard.
- Cupboards for food storage.

Services
Heating

- Recommended temperature 23°C.
- Low temperature heat emitters, maximum surface temperature 43°C.

Hot and cold water

- Hot water delivered at a nominal maximum of 43°C within the band 41–45°C.
- Thermostatic mixers with fail safe devices within 2 m of each hot water outlet.

- Covered hot pipes.
- Cold water (potable).
- Stop valves if required.

Electrics

- Power points for cleaning, bedhead, cooker, microwave, kettle, refrigerator (low level with isolating switch), TV etc.

Systems

- Nurse call with reset and assistance request.
- Smoke detectors.
- Telephone point.
- TV aerial point and video channel.

Environment

Lighting

- Lighting at bedhead and general lighting.
- CIBSE interior lighting code recommended levels: 100 lux bedroom, 150–300 lux kitchenette, 100–300 lux lounge.

Acoustics

- Agreed sound reduction index between rooms (at 40 dB loud speech can be heard but not distinguished; at 45 dB loud speech can be heard faintly but not distinguished; at 50 dB shouting can only be heard with difficulty.

Ventilation

- Fast ventilation required to air room.

Building elements

Windows

- Unobstructed view from bed and armchair.
- No glazing bars at eye level.
- Opening restrictors for first floor windows and above.
- Security for ground floor windows.
- Curtains.

Doors

- 1000 mm wide doors preferred for wheelchair access, and required by some authorities, minimum width 900 mm.

- Identification of individual front doors with photographs, nameplates or colour.

Ironmongery

- Self closers may be required, but are too powerful; automatic hold open devices linked to the fire alarm preferred but expensive.
- Lever handles.
- Lockable doors with emergency lock releases.

(d) Day areas

Location

- Route from day areas to bed-sitting rooms and dining to be as short and free from obstacles as possible.
- Toilets required within close reach.
- Access to secure outside space.
- Small quiet lounges with good access and located where they can be monitored by staff.
- Lounges remote from the main day areas tend not to be used.
- Windows with good or interesting views (service yards are more stimulating to watch than a pretty garden).

User requirements

Residents

- Space for various functions, some not compatible with others (e.g. sitting, conversation, reading, writing, watching the world go by, watching TV, arts, crafts activity, hobbies, workshop, domestic activities, cooking, cleaning, drinks making, gardening, entertaining

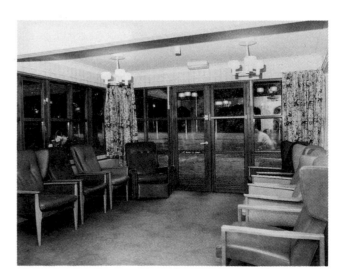

Mall day room with access to garden

visitors, drinking, games, group entertainments, piano playing, religious services, reminiscence therapy, group physiotherapy, dancing, parties).

- Minimum space standards per resident mandatory.
- Small bar required for drinks and snacks dispensing.
- Kitchenette for tea and coffee making.
- Small shop for sweets, cigarettes, toiletries, gifts, cards etc.
- Different furniture arrangements desirable.
- Choice of sitting areas.
- Interesting views.
- Semi-private small conversational groupings if possible.
- Good access.
- Storage for handbags, knitting and personal items.

Care staff
- Good visual supervision.
- Access to all residents.
- Storage for crafts, arts, and hobby equipment, games, books, compact discs, records, tapes, videos, projection equipment etc.

Visitors
- Conversation areas with reasonable privacy.
- Storage space for visiting therapists and other specialists if needed.

Interior
Finishes
- Impervious carpet or non-slip sheet or tile flooring to hobbies areas.
- Domestic decorations, wallpaper and curtains.

Fittings
- Fireplace.
- Fish tank.
- Work surfaces.
- Sinks.
- Bar with small refrigerator, sink, storage.
- Shop counter and storage unit.

Furniture
- High back high seat armchairs.
- Special support chairs.

- Stacking chairs for occasional use.
- Television.
- Sound system or record player.
- Piano or organ.
- Book and display shelves.
- Clock.
- Mirror.
- Pictures.
- Plants.
- Ornaments.
- Sideboard.
- Small tables.
- Footstools.
- Mobile trolleys.
- Tray stands.
- Storage units.

Services
Heating
- Recommended temperature 23°C.
- Low temperature heat emitters, maximum surface temperature 43°C.

Hot and cold water
- Hot water delivered at a nominal maximum of 43°C within the band 41–45°C.
- Thermostatic mixers with fail safe devices within 2 m of each hot water outlet.
- Covered hot pipes.
- Cold water (potable).
- Stop valves may be required.

Electrics
- Power points for cleaning, TV, radio, CD or record player, projection equipment, occasional lighting, tools, equipment.

Systems
- Nurse call with reset and assistance request.
- Smoke detector.
- Fire alarm call points at exits.
- Telephone point or pay phone with reasonable privacy for resident's use.
- TV aerial points and video channel.
- Audio-frequency induction loop system if required.

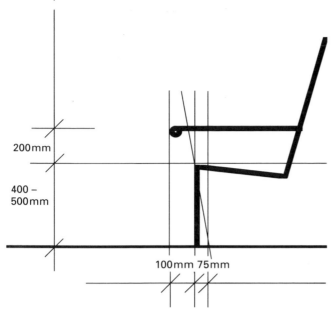

back rest with lumbar and preferably head support

arm rest projecting in front of seat; end of armrest will be used to raise or lower body into seat; must be very stable and give good grip

seat should be warm to touch and not too deep (450mm approx)

clear kick space minimum 75mm back from front of seat

Seating design parameters

Environment

Lighting

- CIBSE interior lighting code recommended levels: lounges 100–300 lux; TV lounges 50 lux; quiet/rest rooms 100 lux.
- Lighting with flattering sideways component.
- High lighting levels.
- No glare or shiny reflective surfaces (CIBSE code limiting glare index 19).
- Dimmer switch if required.
- Emergency lighting.
- Illuminated exit signs.

Acoustics

- Maximize high frequencies.
- Minimize background noise; sound absorption.
- Avoidance of wide columns with acoustic shadows behind them (particularly affecting the high frequencies).
- Avoidance of parallel surfaces of walls and floor/ceiling; use of materials with differing absorbencies.

Building elements

Windows

- Opening lights for quick ventilation.
- Opening restrictors for first floor windows and above.
- No glazing bars at eye level.
- Security for ground floor windows.
- Curtains.

Doors

- 1000 mm wide doors preferred for wheelchair access, and required by some authorities, minimum width 900 mm.
- Unrestricted openings preferred where fire precautions and privacy requirements permit.

Ironmongery

- Self closers may be required, but are too powerful; automatic hold open devices linked to the fire alarm preferred but expensive.
- Lever handles.
- Door and architrave protection to reduce trolley and wheelchair damage.

(e) Hairdressing

Location

- Convenient for day areas; separate room or part of a larger dayroom.
- Away from reception area (most older people enjoy having their hair done but some people with dementia object vociferously to the process).

User requirements

Residents

- Good access.
- High street salon atmosphere.

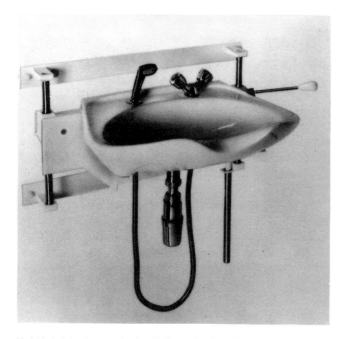

Variable height shampoo basin with Pressalit adjustable height assembly. Height can be adjusted manually or electrically

Hairdresser

- Hair washing sink.
- Styling chair and mirror with all round access.
- Hair dryer and chair if necessary.
- Fixtures suitable for wheelchair users.

Interior

Finishes

- Impervious non-slip vinyl or PVC flooring around wash basin and styling area.
- Splash back to basin.

Fittings

- Hair washing basin with shower attachment.
- Towel rail.
- Large mirror.
- Shelf.
- Cupboard.

Furniture

- Chairs.
- Laundry bin.

Services

Heating

- Recommended temperature 23°C.
- Low temperature heat emitters, maximum surface temperature 43°C.

Hot and cold water

- Hot water delivered at a nominal maximum of 43°C within the band 41–45°C.
- Shower fitting and flexible hose to hairdressing sink
- Thermostatic mixers with fail safe devices within 2 m of each hot water outlet.
- Covered hot pipes.
- Cold water.
- Stop valves if necessary.

Electrics

- Power points for cleaning, dryer, hand dryer and hairdressing equipment used at styling chair.

Systems

- Nurse call with reset and assistance request.
- Smoke detector.

Environment

Lighting

- Lighting with flattering sideways component.
- High lighting levels.
- No glare and shiny reflective surfaces.

Building elements

Windows

- Opening restrictors for first floor windows and above.
- Security for ground floor windows.
- Curtains or blinds.

Doors

- 1000 mm wide doors preferred for wheelchair access, and required by some authorities, minimum width 900 mm.

Ironmongery

- Self closers may be required, but are too powerful; automatic hold open devices linked to the fire alarm preferred but expensive.
- Lever handles.
- Door and architrave protection reduces trolley and wheelchair damage.

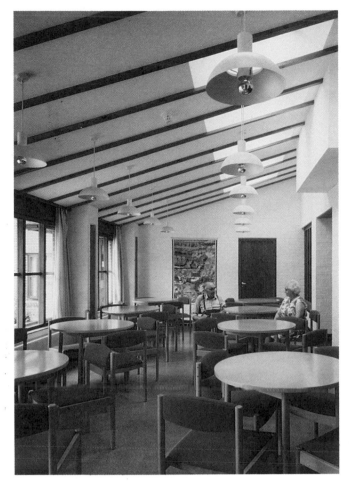

Dining area. Palmer School Road, PRP Architects, 1984

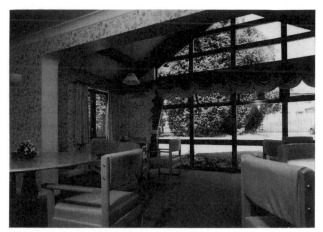

Dining room in a building for confused older people. The dining chairs and tables and domestic curtain and decorations help residents identify the space

(f) Dining areas, restaurant

Location

- Route from dining rooms to bed-sitting rooms and sitting areas to be as short and free from obstacles as possible.
- Toilets within close reach.
- Adjacent to kitchen or with good trolley access; food delivery route separate from dirty linen route.

User requirements

Residents

- Minimum space standards per resident mandatory.
- Tables with four to six places.
- Access for wheelchairs.
- Facilities for those residents not able to eat at a table.
- Homely atmosphere as meals are important events.
- Storage space for hobbies if necessary.
- Flexible arrangements for mealtimes if possible.
- Snack facilities if needed.
- Facilities for visitors to have meals.

Care staff

- Good view of dining areas.
- Access to all residents to assist if needed.
- Food serving space.

Maintenance staff

- Cleanability.

Interior

Finishes

- Impervious carpet or non-slip vinyl or PVC.
- Domestic decorations, wallpaper and curtains.

Furniture

- Tables.
- Chairs.
- Special support chairs for very disabled residents.
- Sideboard for tableware, cutlery and crockery storage.
- Mobile trolleys.
- Tray stands.

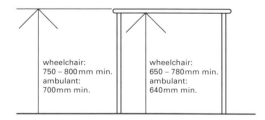

table heights and thigh clearances;
avoid bars at low level; table top should have rounded corners and edges

Table heights

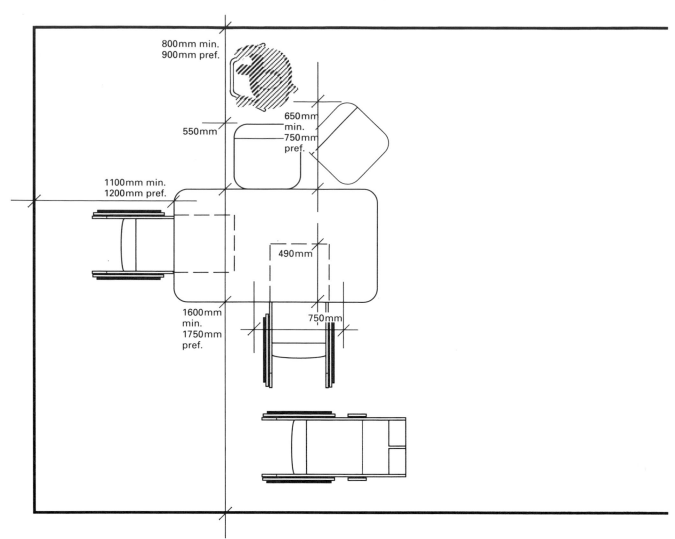

Circulation space around dining tables

Services

Heating

- Temperature 23°C.
- Low temperature heat emitters, maximum surface temperature 43°C.

Electrics

- Power points for cleaning, projection and hobbies equipment.

Systems

- Nurse call with reset and assistance request.
- Smoke detection.
- Telephone point.
- Fire alarm call point by external door.

Environment

Lighting

- CIBSE interior lighting code recommended level 150 lux.
- Flattering modelling techniques.
- High lighting levels.
- No glare and shiny reflective surfaces.
- Emergency lighting.
- Illuminated exit sign.

Acoustics

- Maximize high frequencies.
- Minimize background noise; sound absorption if possible.
- Avoidance of wide columns with acoustic shadows behind them (particularly affecting the high frequencies).
- Avoidance of parallel surfaces of walls and floor/ceiling, use of materials with differing absorbencies as alternative.

Building elements

Windows

- Opening lights for quick ventilation.
- Opening restrictors for first floor windows and above.

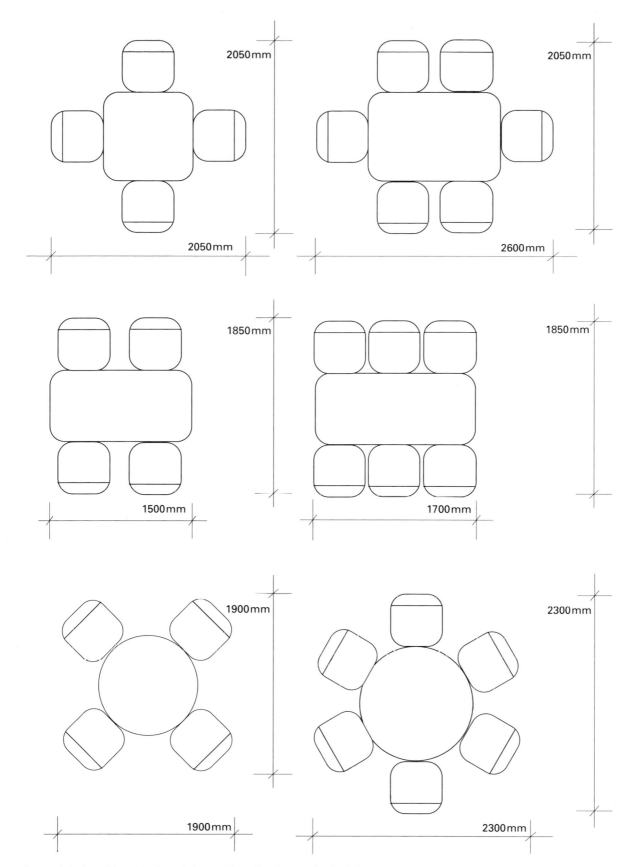

Four- and six-place dining tables for ambulant residents. No allowance for circulation

- Security for ground floor windows if necessary.
- Curtains with blackout linings (if room is to be used for projection).
- No glazing bars at seated eye level.

Doors

- 1000 mm wide doors preferred for wheelchair access, and required by some authorities, minimum width 900 mm.

- Unrestricted openings preferred if fire precautions and privacy requirements permit.

Ironmongery

- Self closers may be required, but are too powerful; automatic hold open devices linked to the fire alarm preferred but expensive.
- Lever handles.
- Door and architrave protection to reduce trolley and wheelchair damage.

(g) Kitchenettes

Location

- Adjacent to day and dining areas.
- Good trolley access to main kitchen; food delivery route separate from dirty linen route.
- Enclosing fire resisting construction if needed (kitchenettes will be regarded as high fire risk areas if used for cooking as well as drinks preparation).

User requirements

Residents

- Preparation of drinks.
- Preparation of light meals or snacks (hygiene regulations prevent residents access to the main kitchen).

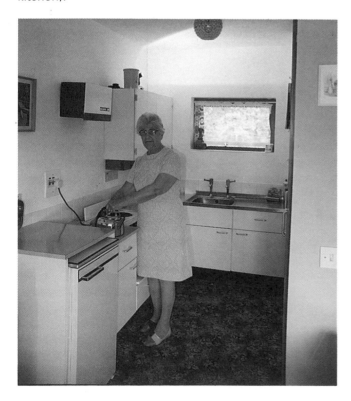

Kitchenette. Liscombe House, PRP Architects, 1976–1977

- Access for wheelchairs.
- Risk of accidental injury or burning to be minimized.

Care staff

- Preparation of drinks.
- Preparation of breakfasts, teas, suppers and snacks.
- Preparation of light meals at night.
- Assisting residents in food preparation.
  Maintenance staff
- Cleanability.

Interior

Finishes

- Non-slip vinyl or PVC flooring with sealed coved skirtings.
- Hygienic wall finish of domestic appearance (check Environmental Health Officer's requirements).
- Impervious non-textured ceiling.

Fittings

- Cooker.
- Microwave.
- Refrigerator.
- Wall and floor cupboards.
- Sink unit.
- Water boiler.
- Work tops.
- Hand wash basin.
- Soap dispenser and hand dryer or towel dispenser and bin.
- Dry powder and BCF fire extinguishers and fire blanket.

Services

Heating

- Recommended temperature 23°C.
- Low temperature heat emitters, maximum surface temperature 43°C.

Hot and cold water

- Hot water delivered at a nominal maximum of 43°C within the band 41–45°C.
- Thermostatic mixers with fail safe devices within 2 m of each hot water outlet.
- Covered hot pipes.

- Cold water (potable).
- Stop valves if necessary.

Mechanical ventilation
- Extract fan or cooker hood.

Electrics
- Power points remote from sink for cleaning, refrigerator (low level with isolator switch), water boiler, kettle and kitchen equipment.
- Pull cord to light.

Systems
- Nurse call with reset and assistance request.
- Smoke and or heat detection.
- Fire alarm call point by external door.

Environment
Lighting
- CIBSE interior lighting code recommended level 150–300 lux.
- No shadows on work surfaces.
- Emergency lighting.
- Illuminated exit sign.
- Washable luminaire.

Building elements
Windows
- Opening lights for quick ventilation.
- Opening restrictors required for first floor windows and above.
- Security for ground floor windows if necessary.
- Blinds.

Doors
- 1000 mm wide doors preferred for wheelchair access, and required by some authorities; minimum width 900 mm.
- Worktop height gate if necessary to restrict access.
- Hatch to dining area if necessary (it will need to be fire resistant and self closing).

Ironmongery
- Self closers if necessary.
- Lever handles.

- Door and architrave protection to reduce trolley and wheelchair damage.

2.2.3 Residents' ablutions
(a) Bathing
Location
- Near day areas and bed-sitting rooms (bathroom equipped with a hoist or a special bath will be heavily used).
- Remote from main entrance and public areas (some demented residents dislike bathing and can be noisy).

User requirements
Residents
- Curtains or screen if necessary (privacy and dignity must be maintained; it should not be possible to see someone in the bath if the door is left open).
- Homely decorations and lighting (special baths and hoists are intimidating).
- Seat.
- Toilet.
- Robust fittings and fixings (items fixed to walls will be used for support).
- Minimum space standards if necessary.
- Minimum provision mandatory.

Care staff
- Special or raised baths or hoists (back injuries are caused by bending and lifting).
- Space for helper on each side of resident bathing.

Maintenance staff
- Ducted services and coved skirtings for easy cleaning.
- Drains with good rodding access.

Interior
Finishes
- Non-slip vinyl or PVC flooring.
- Coved skirtings sealed to walls.
- Hygienic splash and steam-proof surfaces.
- Homely rather than clinical decorations.

Fittings
- Bath (1.7 m, 1.5 m or special assisted) with flat non-slip base.

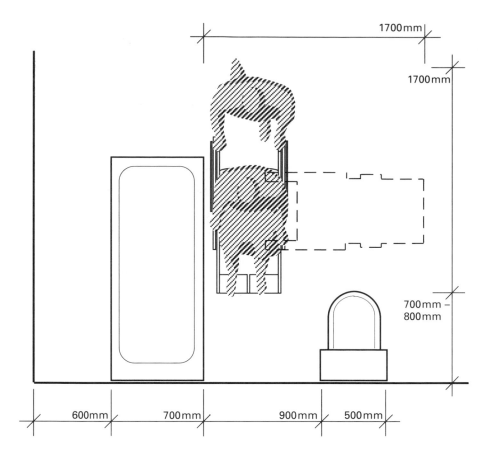

1700mm

1700mm

700mm – 800mm

600mm   700mm   900mm   500mm

Wheelchair turning space within bathroom

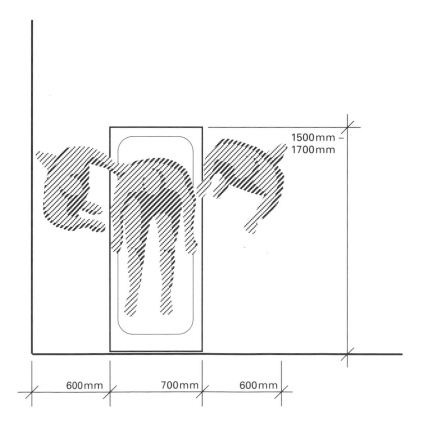

1500mm – 1700mm

600mm   700mm   600mm

Assisted bathing

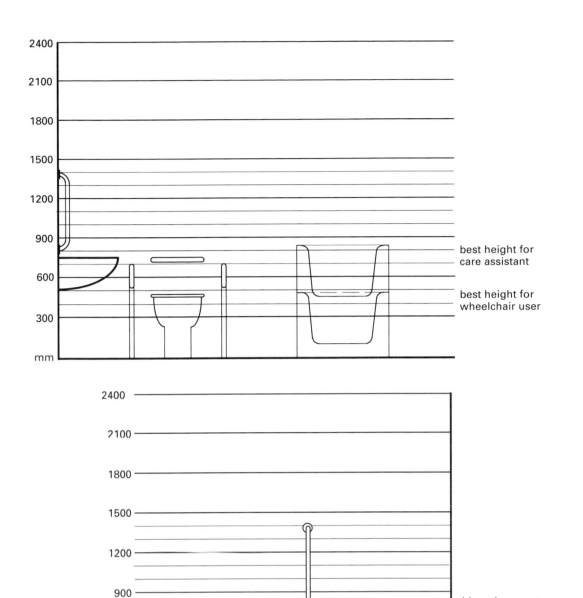

best height for
care assistant

best height for
wheelchair user

hinged support
rails will be heavily
loaded; robust
wall fittings are
needed

Fixing heights of bathroom fittings and grab rails

- Hoist or lifting aid.
- Toilet.
- Toilet roll holder.
- Grab rails (vertical, horizontal, cranked and drop down).
- Wash hand basin.
- Lever or cross top taps.
- Thermostatic mixer controls.
- Shower.
- Towel rail (will be used as grab rail).
- Soap dish.

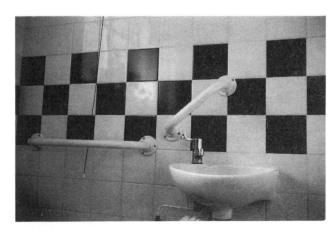

Grab rail mounted at 45° over wash hand basin

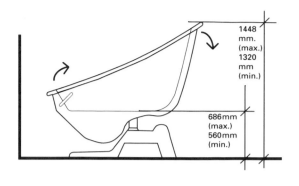

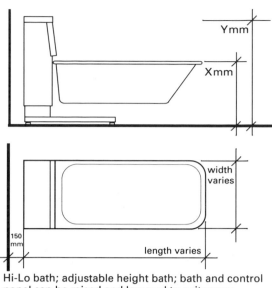

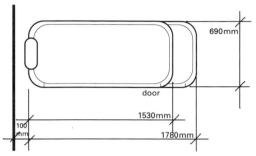

Hi-Lo bath; adjustable height bath; bath and control panel can be raised and lowered to suit users; several sizes available

Parker bath; height adjustment by electric or foot operated hydraulic pump; door on left hand side only

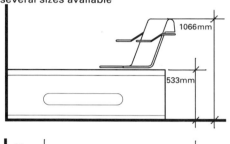

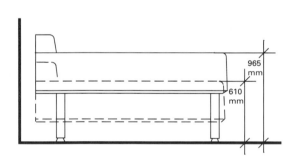

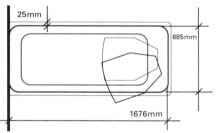

Solo bath; bath has swivelling height adjustable seat

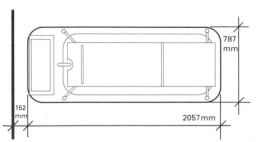

elevating Madison bath; adjustable height bath shown with optional bathing table; bath can be raised and lowered to suit users; fixed height version set at 838mm available

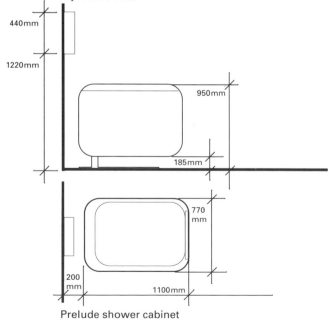

Prelude shower cabinet

Specialist baths and shower

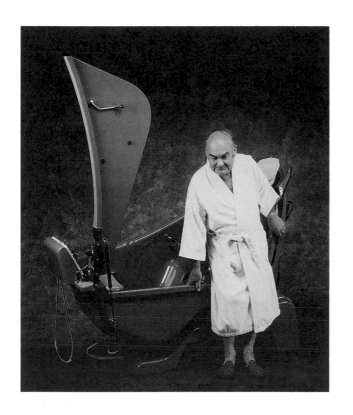
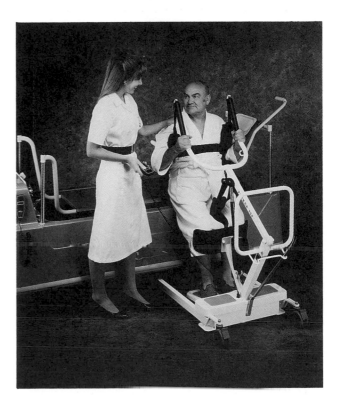
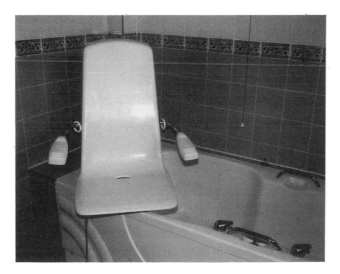
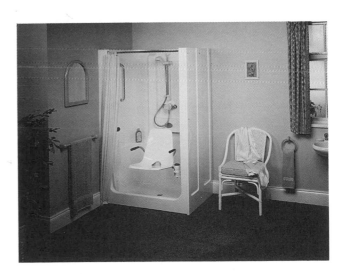

Top left. Parker bath. (Reproduced with permission from Parker Bath Company Ltd.)

Top right. Madison bath. (Reproduced with permission from Parker Bath Company Ltd.)

Bottom left. Bath with swivel seat

Bottom right. Parker Dignity shower. (Reproduced with permission from Parker Bath Company Ltd.)

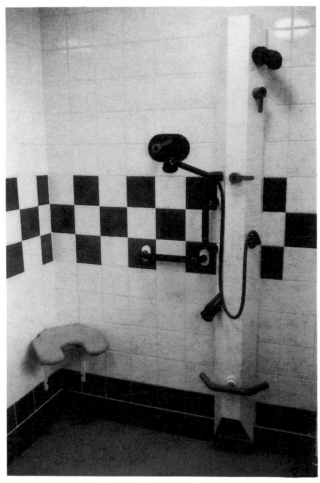

Above. Shower with three shower heads for use in standing, sitting or for foot washing

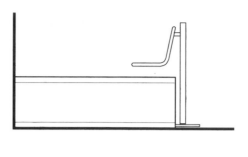

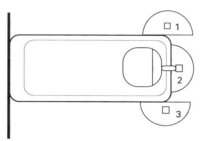

static ambulift: fixed hand operated lift; baseplate may be mounted in three positions; must be securely bolted to a concrete base

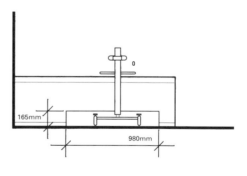

165mm

980mm

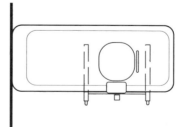

small mobile hoist; cut out required in panelled baths to accommodate wheels, or baths may be raised; dimensions shown suit the Arjo mobile hoist; clearance required should be checked with hoist supplier

Left and above. Hoists and lifting aids

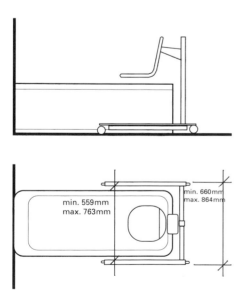

min. 660mm
max. 864mm

min. 559mm
max. 763mm

mobile ambulift: a mobile lift with adjustable chassis legs; lift can be adapted for a chair or a sling

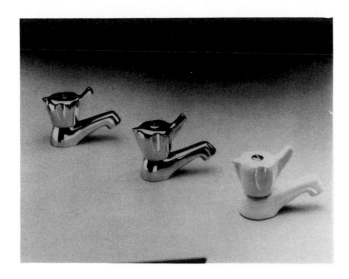

- Soap dispenser for staff.
- Hand dryer for staff or towel dispenser.
- Hat and coat hooks.
- Toothbrush holder.
- Shelf for toilet bag, denture glass, talcum powder, hairbrush and comb.
- Mirror.
- Shaver point and mirror light.

Furniture
- Chair.
- Bin.

Services

Heating
- Recommended temperature 23°C.
- Low temperature heat emitters, maximum surface temperature 43°C.

Hot and cold water
- Hot water delivered at a nominal maximum of 43°C within the band 41–45°C or maximum 37–38°C for bidets.
- Covered hot pipes, maximum surface temperature 43°C.
- Thermostatic mixers with fail safe devices within 2 m of each hot water outlet.
- Cold water (potable) to wash basin.
- Stop valves if necessary.

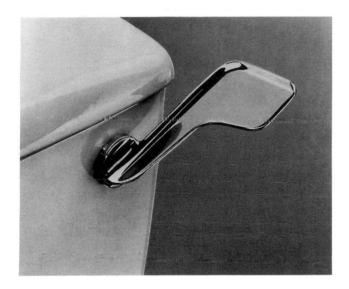

Drainage
- Rodding access.

Mechanical ventilation
- Ventilation minimum extract rate 15 litre/second, operated intermittently if necessary.

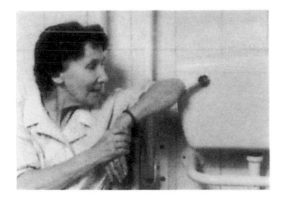

Electrics
- Pull cords to switches.

Systems
- Nurse call cord between bath and toilet of different colour to light pull cords.

Top. Novaturn taps and mixers. Taps have handwheels with raised lobe and thumb grip, and are suitable for people with weak or arthritic hands. (Reproduced with permission from Phlexicare, Nicholls and Clarke Ltd.)

Middle and bottom. Spatulate cistern lever. The lever is easy to grip, or can be operated with clenched fist or elbow. It can be adapted to fit most cisterns. (Reproduced with permission from Phlexicare, Nicholls and Clarke Ltd.)

Environment

Lighting

- CIBSE interior lighting code recommended level 150 lux.
- Shaver light at mirror with pull cord.
- Moisture-resistant luminaires.

Acoustics

- Sound reduction if necessary.

Building elements

Windows

- Obscured glass.
- Opening restrictors for upper floor windows.
- Opening light for quick ventilation.
- Security for ground floor windows.
- Curtain or blind.

Floors

- Hoists and lifting aids fixed to concrete base if necessary.

Doors

- Positioned so that bath is not seen.
- 1000 mm wide doors preferred for wheelchair access, and required by some authorities, minimum width 900 mm.

Ironmongery

- Indicator bolt with emergency release openable from outside.
- Kick plates and door protection to prevent damage by hoist and wheelchairs.
- Lever handles.

(b) Residents' toilets

Location

- Adjacent to dayrooms and dining areas.
- Within reach of bed-sitting rooms (12 m maximum distance from bed-sitting rooms required by some registering authorities).
- Provision of toilets in bathrooms desirable.
- En-suite with some or all bed-sitting rooms.
- Accessible to outside seating areas.
- Separate facilities for staff, visitors and kitchen staff.

User requirements

Residents

- Privacy and dignity to be maintained (it should not be possible to see someone on the toilet if the door is left open).
- Robust fittings and fixings (items fixed to walls will be used for support).
- Ability to lock door from a wheelchair.
- Minimum space standards if necessary.
- Minimum provision mandatory.

Care staff

- Space for helper on each side of some residents (at least around toilets in frequent use).
- Separate facilities for staff.

Maintenance staff

- Ducted services and coved skirtings for easy cleaning.
- Drains with rodding access.

Interior

Finishes

- Non-slip vinyl or PVC floors.
- Coved skirtings sealed to walls and fittings.
- Hygienic surfaces.

Fittings

- Toilet seat height recommended for wheelchair users: 480 mm; for semi-ambulant users: 430 mm; best height for comfortable use: 380 mm (detachable seat raisers or footstools may be required).
- Backrest desirable.
- Bolt-down cistern and heavy duty seats needed for some residents.
- Grab rails (vertical, horizontal, cranked, drop down).
- Wash hand basin.
- Lever or cross top taps.
- Thermostatic mixer controls.
- Toilet roll holder.
- Towel rail in en-suite bathroom.
- Soap dish in en-suite bathroom.
- Toothbrush holder in en-suite bathroom.
- Shelf for toilet bag, denture glass, talcum powder, hairbrush and comb in en-suite bathroom.
- Mirror.

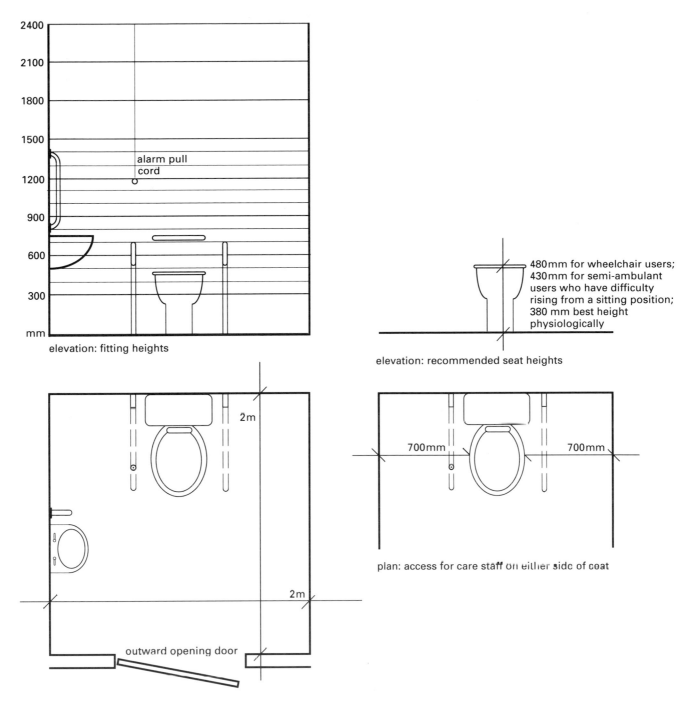

elevation: fitting heights

480 mm for wheelchair users; 430 mm for semi-ambulant users who have difficulty rising from a sitting position; 380 mm best height physiologically

elevation: recommended seat heights

plan: assisted toilet: space for care assistant on either side of resident

plan: access for care staff on either side of coat

Residents' toilet dimensions

- Shaver point and mirror light.
- Soap dispenser.
- Hand dryer or towel dispenser and bin.

Services

Heating

- Recommended temperature 21°C.

Hot and cold water

- Hot water delivered at a nominal maximum of 43°C within the band 41–45°C.
- Thermostatic mixers with fail safe devices within 2 m of each hot water outlet.
- Covered hot pipes, maximum surface temperature 43°C.
- Cold water (potable to wash basin in en-suite bathroom).

- Cisterns to internal toilets with tundish overflows if necessary, with approval of water authority.
- Stop valves if necessary.

Drainage
- Good rodding access.

Mechanical ventilation
- Ventilation minimum three air changes per hour (operated intermittently if necessary, with 15 minutes overrun, or one or more ventilation openings with a total area of at least 1/20th floor area and with some part of the ventilation opening at least 1.75 m above the floor level).

Electrics
- Pull cord light fitting distinguishable from nurse call pull cord.

Systems
- Nurse call pull cord adjacent to toilet.
- Room presence indicator if necessary.

Environment
Lighting
- CIBSE interior lighting code recommended level 100 lux.
- Mirror light with pull cord.

Acoustics
- Sound reduction if necessary.

Building elements
Windows
- Obscured glass.
- Opening light for quick ventilation.
- Opening restrictors to upper floor windows.
- Security for ground floor windows.
- Curtain or blind.

Doors
- Outward opening or double swing doors (to enable staff to reach someone collapsed inside the room).
- 1000 mm wide doors preferred for wheelchair access, and required by some authorities,

minimum width 900 mm.

Ironmongery
- Indicator bolt with emergency release.
- Kick plate to prevent damage by wheelchairs.
- Lever handles.
- Clear pictogram or nameplate to aid identification of room by residents.

2.2.4 Residents' care
(a) Nurse station
Location
- Good but discrete visual supervision of the main day or night areas.

User requirements
Care staff
- Handover meetings at shift changes.
- Secure records storage.
- Nurse call system monitoring.
- Note writing.
- A degree of privacy from residents desirable.

Interior
Finishes
- Impervious carpet.
- Domestic decorations.

Fittings
- Worktop.
- Notice board.

Furniture
- Desk.
- Filing cabinet.
- Chairs.

Services
Heating
- Recommended temperature 21°C.
- Low temperature heat emitters, maximum surface temperature 43°C.

Electrics
- Power points for cleaning and office equipment.

Systems

- Nurse call main panel or monitoring panel.
- Smoke detection.
- Telephone point.

Doors

- Gate to restrict access by residents if necessary.

(b) Sluice, dirty utility
Location

- Accessible to bed-sitting rooms and laundry or soiled linen collection point.
- Sluice on each floor.
- Dirty linen route around building to be separate from food delivery route if required by local authority (precautions need to be taken to ensure there is no risk of cross-infection from handling dirty linen and food).
- Inter-floor connection to laundry by chute if necessary.
- Stores or toilets to form sound buffers between sluice rooms with automatic equipment and bed-sitting rooms.

User requirements
Care staff

- Disposal of faecal matter from soiled sheets, clothing or bed pans.
- Cleansing of soiled bed pans and commodes.
- Initial cleansing and bagging of soiled sheets and clothing.
- Automatic sluicing of sheets and clothing.
- Automatic washing of bed pans.
- Storage of bed pans and urine bottles.
- Hand washing.
- Good working environment.

Maintenance staff

- Hygienic and easily cleaned finishes.

Interior
Finishes

- Non-slip vinyl or tile.
- Glazed tiling or other impervious finish.

Fittings

- Belfast sink and drainer.
- Slop hopper.
- Bed pan washer/slop sink.
- Automatic sluicing machine.
- Automatic bed pan washing machine.
- Wash hand basin.
- Soap dispenser.
- Hand dryers or paper towel dispensers.
- Shelving.

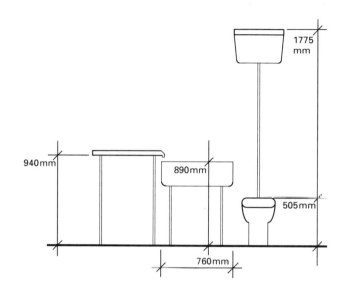

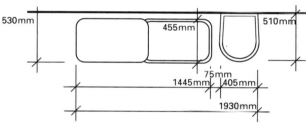

slop hopper and sink combination:
all or part of the combination may be specified

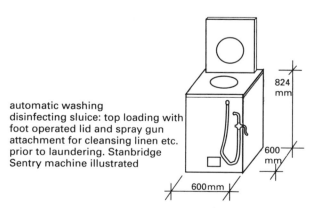

automatic washing disinfecting sluice: top loading with foot operated lid and spray gun attachment for cleansing linen etc. prior to laundering. Stanbridge Sentry machine illustrated

Manual and automatic sluices

Furniture
- Waste bin.
- Soiled linen bin.

Services
Heating
- Recommended temperature 18°C.

Hot and cold water
- Hot and cold water to wash basin sink and slop hopper or bed pan washer.
- Cold and possibly hot feed to automatic machines (pressure may need boosting).
- Stop valves.

Drainage
- Slop hoppers, sluices and bed pan washers are soil appliances.
- Rodding access.

Mechanical ventilation
- Extract fan.

Electrics
- 3-phase supply for automatic sluice or bed pan washers if necessary.
- Pull cord to light switch.

Systems
- Smoke detection where mechanical equipment installed.

Environment
Lighting
- CIBSE interior lighting code recommended level 150 lux.

Acoustics
- Sound proofing if necessary.

Building elements
Windows
- Security for ground floor windows if necessary.
- Obscured glass.

Floors
- Special floor fixing for some automatic machines to dampen vibration (not all floors are suitable).

Doors
- Outward opening or double swing doors if necessary for easier access by staff with their hands full.
- Camouflaged doors by use of wall finish to deter confused residents from entering.

Ironmongery
- Lever handles or pull handle and push plate.

(c) Treatment, clean utility, drug store
Location
- Secure location in a well overlooked position.
- Good access for drugs trolley to day areas.

User requirements
Care staff
- Storage, preparation and distribution of drugs.
- Storage of clinical equipment.
- Possible use for treatment of minor injuries or chiropody (medical examinations normally take place in the resident's room).

Interior
Finishes
- Non-slip vinyl or tile, coved skirtings sealed to wall.
- Glazed tiling or other impervious finish.

Fittings
- Sink unit.
- Wall and floor cupboards with lockable doors.
- Hand rinse basin.
- Soap dispenser.
- Hand dryer or paper towel dispenser and bin.
- Shelving.
- Worktop.
- Refrigerator.
- Locked drugs cupboard securely fixed to wall or floor.
- Drugs trolley with chain fixing to wall.
- Notice board.

Furniture

- Clinical waste bin.
- Treatment seat or couch.
- Stool.
- Desk and chair.

Services

Heating

- Temperature 23°C if used for treatment, otherwise 21°C.
- Low temperature heat emitters, maximum surface temperature 43°C.

Hot and cold water

- Hot water delivered at a nominal maximum of 43°C within the band 41–45°C.
- Thermostatic mixers with fail safe devices within 2 m of each hot water outlet.
- Covered hot pipes.
- Cold water (potable).
- Stop valves if necessary.

Drainage

- Drainage to sink unit and wash hand basin.

Electrics

- Extract fan.
- Power points for cleaning, refrigerator (low level with isolating switch) plus twin socket for general use.

Systems

- Drugs cupboard door connected to nurse call system or warning light outside room door.
- Smoke detector.

Environment

Lighting

- CIBSE interior lighting code recommended level 300 lux for medical inspection lamp at couch position where room used for treatment, otherwise 150 lux.

Building elements

Windows

- Rooms without windows for security.
- Additional security for windows if required.

- Obscured glass.
- Blinds.

Walls

- Masonry wall or specially strengthened wall if necessary for fixing drugs trolley.

Floors

- Non-slip vinyl, PVC or tile.

Doors

- Doors camouflaged by use of wall finish to deter confused residents from entering.

Ironmongery

- Lockable door.
- Door and architrave protection to prevent damage by trolleys.

2.2.5 Storage

(a) Linen

Location

- Accessible to bed-sitting rooms and laundry.
- Storage areas best located near bed-sitting rooms.
- Stores on external walls for passive ventilation.
- Holding store for soiled linen near service entrance where laundry is contracted out.

User requirements

Care staff

- Accessible shelving.

Interior

Finishes

- Carpet or vinyl.
- Emulsion paint.

Fittings

- Slatted shelving 300 mm deep for sheets and 450 mm deep for duvets; highest stored item at 1650 mm above floor level.

Services

Electrics

- Power point for cleaning.

Systems

- Smoke detector.

Environment

Lighting

- CIBSE interior lighting code recommended level 100 lux.

Ventilation

- Some air movement desirable.

Building elements

Doors

- Outward opening or double swing doors if necessary for easier access by staff with their hands full.
- Camouflaged doors with wall finish to deter confused residents from entering.

Ironmongery

- Lockable door.

(b) Wheelchairs

Location

- Accessible to main entrance and dayrooms.

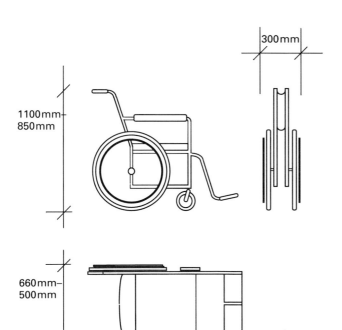

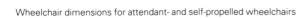

Wheelchair dimensions for attendant- and self-propelled wheelchairs

User requirements

Management

- Decision on number of wheelchairs to be stored (options: allow residents to bring their own wheelchairs or provide a small number of chairs for general use).

Care staff

- Accessible.

Maintenance staff

- Easy to clean.

Interior

Finishes

- Emulsion paint.

Electrics

- Power point for cleaning.

Systems

- Smoke detector.

Environment

Lighting

- CIBSE interior lighting code recommended level 100 lux.

Ventilation

- Passive ventilation to outside air.

Building elements

Doors

- Door and architrave protection to prevent damage.

Walls

- Wall protection to prevent damage.

Ironmongery

- Lockable door.

(c) Equipment

Location

- Accessible to bed-sitting rooms, bathrooms and dayrooms.

User requirements
Care staff

- Accessible.
- Storage for hoists and lifting equipment, walking aids.
- Storage for crockery and cutlery and tableware.
- Storage for day area resources.
- Storage for equipment used by visiting therapists and other specialists.

Interior
Finishes

- Emulsion paint.

Fittings

- Shelving: highest convenient shelf for items in regular use at 1650 mm above floor level.
- Floor space for tall items.

Services
Electrics

- Power point for cleaning.

Systems

- Smoke detector.

Environment
Lighting

- CIBSE interior lighting code recommended level 100 lux.

Building elements
Doors

- Doors can be camouflaged by using wall finish to deter confused residents from entering.

Ironmongery

- Lockable doors.

(d) Long-term storage
User requirements
Maintenance staff

- Safe access for long-term storage.
- Storage for hoists, lifting equipment and walking aids.
- Storage for suitcases and spare bedroom furniture (where residents are encouraged to furnish their own rooms).

Interior
Finishes

- Dust-resistant.

Fittings

- Shelving.
- Floor space for tall items.

Services
Heating

- Frost-free.

Electrics

- Power point for cleaning.

Systems

- Smoke detector with indicator light.

Environment
Lighting

- CIBSE interior lighting code recommended level 100 lux.

Building elements
Doors

- Camouflaged doors with wall finish to deter confused residents from entering.

Ironmongery

- Lockable doors.

(e) Continence aids
Location

- Accessible to bed-sitting rooms and bathrooms.

User requirements
Care staff

- Accessible.

Interior
Finishes

- Emulsion paint.

Fittings

- Shelving: highest convenient shelf for items in regular use at 1650 mm above floor level.

Services
Electrics
- Power point for cleaning.

Systems
- Smoke detector.

Building elements
Ironmongery
- Lockable doors.

(f) Cleaning equipment
Location
- Cleaner's store on each floor if possible (organic stains need to be removed quickly to prevent odours developing).
- No access to residents (cleaners' stores contain dangerous substances).

User requirements
Maintenance staff
- Accessible shelving.
- Filling and emptying of buckets.
- Storage of upright cleaners, mops and brooms and cleaning materials.

Interior
Finishes
- Non-slip vinyl or tile floor.
- Emulsion paint and tile splash back to sink.

Fittings
- Washable shelving 250 mm deep for cleaning materials: highest shelf for items in regular use at 1650 mm above floor level.
- Bucket sink and grating.

Services
Electrics
- Power point for cleaning.

Mechanical ventilation
- Extract fan.

Systems
- Smoke detector.

Environment
Lighting
- CIBSE interior lighting code recommended level 100 lux.

Building elements
Doors
- Outward opening door if necessary for easier access by staff with their hands full.
- Camouflaged door with wall finish to deter confused residents from entering.

Ironmongery
- Lockable door.

2.2.6 Administration
(a) Administration areas
Location
- Near main entrance.
- Combined with reception of visitors if required.

User requirements
Administrative staff
- Monitoring of visitors.
- Secure records storage.
- Administration of home.
- Private interviews and meetings.
- Telephone reception.

Visitors
- Reception and welcome.
- Private interviews with manager or staff.

Interior
Finishes
- Impervious carpet.
- Good standard of decoration (visitors get first impression of home here).

Fittings
- Shelving.
- Reception desk or hatch.
- Notice board.

Furniture
- Desk.

- Typist's chair.
- Filing cabinets with locks.
- Easy chairs.
- Coffee table.

Services
Heating
- Recommended temperature 23°C.
- Low temperature heat emitters, maximum surface temperature 43°C.

Electrics
- Power points for cleaning, plus twin sockets for office equipment and general use.

Systems
- Telephone main panel.
- Monitored line to call emergency services.
- Nurse call main panel or slave panel.
- Security monitor.
- Smoke detectors.

Environment
Lighting
- CIBSE interior lighting code recommended levels: offices and enquiry desks 500 lux limiting glare index 19 (could be localized lighting).

Acoustics
- Sound proofing to private interview space.

Building elements
Windows
- Additional security for windows if necessary.
- Curtains or blinds.

Ironmongery
- Lockable door to office.

(b) Visitors' toilets
Location
- Adjacent to entrance.

User requirements
Visitors
- Designed to ambulant disabled standards (many of the visitors will be as old as the residents).
- Robust fittings and fixings (items fixed to walls will be used for support).
- Cloaks hanging space if necessary.
- Provision mandatory in some cases.

Maintenance staff
- Ducted services and coved skirtings for easy cleaning.
- Rodding access to drains.

Interior
Finishes
- Non-slip vinyl or PVC floors.
- Coved skirtings sealed to walls and fittings.
- Hygienic surfaces.

Fittings
- Wash hand basin.
- Grab rails (vertical, horizontal, cranked).
- Lever or cross top taps.
- Thermostatic mixer controls.
- Toilet roll holder.
- Shelf for handbag.
- Mirror.
- Soap dispenser.
- Hand dryer or towel dispenser and bin.
- Hat and coat hooks.

Services
Heating
- Recommended temperature 21°C.

Hot and cold water
- Hot water delivered at a nominal maximum of 43°C within the band 41–45°C.
- Thermostatic mixers with fail safe devices within 2 m of each hot water outlet.
- Covered hot pipes, maximum surface temperature 43°C.
- Cold water.
- Cisterns to internal toilets with tundish overflows if necessary, with approval of water authority.
- Stop valves if necessary.

Drainage
- Good rodding access.

Mechanical ventilation

- Ventilation minimum three air changes per hour (operated intermittently if necessary, with 15 minutes overrun or one or more ventilation openings with a total area of at least 1/20th floor area and with some part of the ventilation opening at least 1.75 m above the floor level).

Electrics

- Pull cord light fitting.

Environment

Lighting

- CIBSE interior lighting code recommended level 100 lux.

Acoustics

- Sound reduction if necessary.

Building elements

Windows

- Obscured glass.
- Opening light for quick ventilation.
- Security for ground floor windows.
- Curtain or blind.

Doors

- Minimum width 900 mm.

Ironmongery

- Indicator bolt with emergency release.
- Kick plate to prevent damage by wheelchairs.
- Lever handles.
- Pictogram or nameplate.

(c) Staff rooms

Location

- Accessible to residents' spaces in emergencies.

User requirements

Care staff

- Rest periods.
- Meal and drinks breaks.
- Snack preparation.
- Shift change meetings.

- Meetings.
- Seminars.
- Training sessions.
- Exchange of information.
- Smoking or not depending on home policy.

Interior

Finishes

- Carpet or vinyl, PVC or tile (waterproof area around sink unit).
- Splash back to sink unit.

Fittings

- Sink unit, refrigerator, microwave and worktop.
- Notice board.
- Lockers.
- Dry powder fire extinguisher.

Furniture

- Chairs.
- Tables.

Services

Heating

- Recommended temperature 21°C.

Hot and cold water

- Hot and cold (potable) water to sink unit.

Drainage

- To sink unit.

Electrics

- Power points for cleaning, refrigerator (low level with isolating switch), kettle, microwave, projection equipment.

Systems

- Nurse call slave panel.
- Smoke detection.
- Fire alarm call point at exit.

Environment

Lighting

- CIBSE interior lighting code recommended level 100 lux.

- Emergency lighting.
- Illuminated exit sign to external door.

Building elements
Windows
- Security for ground floor windows if necessary.
- Curtains or blinds.

Ironmongery
- Lockable door.

(d) Staff cloaks, shower and toilets
Location
- Near staff room.

User requirements
Care staff
- Health and Safety at Work Act 1974 provisions.
- Secure storage of coats and handbags.
- Changing clothes.
- Washing and showering.
- Combing hair, doing make-up.
- Toilets not shared with residents or kitchen staff.
- Separate changing and toilet facilities for male and female staff.

Interior
Finishes
- Non-slip vinyl, PVC or tile, sealed and coved skirtings.
- Tiling to shower and splash backs to sanitary fittings.
- Water-resistant finishes.

Fittings
- Mirrors.
- Handbag shelf.
- Hat and coat hooks.
- Lockers.
- Shoe storage.
- Shower.
- Shower seat.
- Shower cubicle.
- Male and female toilets.
- Toilet roll holder.
- Sanitary protection disposal unit.
- Wash hand basins.

- Taps.
- Soap dispenser and hand drying facilities.

Furniture
- Bin.
- Chair.

Services
Heating
- Recommended temperature 18–21°C.

Hot and cold water
- Hot and cold water to shower, wash hand basins; cold water to toilets; thermostatic control to shower.
- Stop valves if necessary.

Drainage
- To shower, wash hand basins and toilets.
- Rodding access.

Mechanical ventilation
- To shower and toilets.

Electrics
- Pull cords to light switches.

Systems
- Smoke detection.

Environment
Lighting
- CIBSE interior lighting code recommended level 100 lux.
- Emergency lighting.
- Light fitting with shaver point over mirror.

Acoustics
- Sound reduction to toilets.

Building elements
Windows
- Obscured glass.
- Curtain or blind.
- Security for ground floor windows if necessary.

Ironmongery
- Bathroom locks with indicator bolts.

2.2.7 Kitchen and laundry

(a) Kitchen

Food preparation may be done on the premises or by outside caterers. Where caterers are used, a food reception area and regeneration equipment will be required. Catering kitchens are normally designed and installed by specialists. The broad requirements are:

Location
- Good access for delivery vehicles and refuse collection.
- Kitchen service yard non-obvious to visitors (although it is of interest to residents).
- Convenient food delivery route to dining areas.
- Separate kitchen and food delivery route from laundry and soiled linen route (to prevent cross-infection; other methods may be acceptable if the routes merge).
- Access to toilet for exclusive use of kitchen staff.

User requirements
Management
- Prevention of petty theft.

Kitchen staff
- Space for administration: ordering, telephone, accounts, menu preparation, notice board.
- Regeneration ovens where outside caterers are used.
- Food storage.
- Equipment storage.
- Vegetable washing and preparation.
- Meal preparation.
- Drinks preparation.
- Cooking.
- Waste disposal.
- Servery.
- Pan wash.
- Wash up.
- Crockery and cutlery storage.
- Cleaning.
- First aid.

- Access to cloaks space, lockers and exclusive use of toilet.

Interior
Finishes
- Non-slip impervious easy-clean floor.
- Full height wall tiling or other impervious hygienic wall finish with sealed coved skirtings (check Environmental Health Officer's requirements).
- Impervious non-textured ceiling finish.

Fittings
- Refrigerator.
- Freezer.
- Washable shelving.
- Vegetable preparation sink.
- Work tops.
- Preparation sinks.
- Wash hand basin.
- Soap dispenser and hand dryer or towel dispenser and bin.
- Cooking range.
- Extract fan and hood over cooking range.
- Food preparation equipment.
- Water boiler.
- Wash up sinks and drainers.
- Dish washer.
- Hot cupboards.
- Storage racking.
- Shelving.
- Notice board.
- BCF and dry powder fire extinguishers.
- Fire blanket.

Furniture
- Chairs.
- Desk.

Services
Heating
- Recommended temperature 18°C.

Hot and cold water
- Hot and cold (potable) to sinks and hand basin.
- Stop valves.

Drainage
- To sinks, hand basin, dish washer.
- Capped off drain connection in suitable position for future expansion of installation.
- Rodding access.

Mechanical ventilation
- Extraction over cooking range.

Electrics
- Power points for cleaning.
- 3-phase supply for catering equipment.
- Power points to suit layout.

Gas
- Gas supply to gas-fired installations.

Systems
- Smoke and or heat detectors.
- Fire alarm call point.
- Telephone point.
- Intercom.

Environment
Lighting
- CIBSE interior lighting code recommended levels: food preparation and cooking areas: 500 lux; stores: 150 lux; servery, vegetable preparation and washing up areas: 300 lux.
- No shadows on working areas.
- Washable luminaires.
- Emergency lighting.
- Illuminated exit sign.

Acoustics
- Sound absorption if necessary.

Ventilation
- Additional fast ventilation to lower temperature or dispel steam.
- Vermin-proof ventilation to food stores.

Building elements
Windows
- Opening lights need fixed fly screens.
- Security for ground floor windows.

Wall/roof
- Flue and cowl to extract fan to be indicated on planning application drawings.

Doors
- Wide doors preferred for trolley access, minimum width 900 mm.
- Door and architrave protection to minimize damage by trolleys.
- Vision panel.

Ironmongery
- Lockable doors to stores.

(b) Laundry
Good laundering and ironing facilities are essential so that residents look well turned out. Laundry may be partly or entirely contracted out or done on the premises. Note that machine noise and vibration could cause problems in adjacent rooms and floors.

Location
- Convenient for linen collection from bed-sitting rooms.
- Separate from kitchen, dining and meal delivery route.
- Access to secure outside drying space if necessary.
- Ventilation ducts for dryers to outside wall.
- Storage area for dirty linen near service entrance if laundry is contracted out.

User requirements
Residents
- Risk of cross-contamination from soiled linen to be eliminated.
- Provision for residents to do their own washing if necessary in residential homes.

Maintenance staff
- Good working conditions.
- Separate clean and dirty work areas (there should be a linear progression through the laundry with soiled linen entering at one end and clean leaving at the other; where there is a high risk of infection special

washing machines with separate doors for loading and unloading are available).

Interior

Finishes

- Non-slip vinyl or quarry tile with coved skirtings sealed to wall.
- Wall tiling, gloss, eggshell or silk vinyl emulsion paint.
- Splash backs to sink and hand basin.

Fittings

- Industrial or commercial washing machines (domestic machines are not recommended except where provided for resident's own use).
- Washer with sluice cycle.
- Dryers.
- Spin dryers.
- Drying cupboard.
- Airing cupboard.
- Sink unit.
- Wash hand basin.
- Soap dispenser and hand dryer or towel dispenser and bin.
- Worktop.
- Rotary iron.
- Racking and shelving.
- Dirty linen bin.
- Notice board.

Furniture

- Ironing board and iron.

Services

Heating

- Recommended temperature 18°C.

Hot and cold water

- Hot and cold supplies to sinks and wash hand basins; cold and/or hot supplies to machines (pressure booster pump may be required).
- Stop valves.

Drainage

- To machines, sink and wash hand basin.
- Rodding access.

Mechanical ventilation

- Extract fan.
- Dryers to be ventilated via duct to open air.

Electrics

- Power points for cleaning and ironing.
- 3-phase supply for machines.
- Pull cord to light switch.

Gas

- To gas-powered equipment.

Systems

- Smoke or heat detector.
- Fire alarm call point at external door.
- Telephone point or intercom.

Environment

Lighting

- CIBSE interior lighting code recommended level for laundries 300 lux.
- Emergency lighting.
- Illuminated exit sign.

Acoustics

- Sound absorption or buffers (machines can be noisy).

Ventilation

- Ventilation to outside air required where gas laundry equipment installed.

Building elements

Windows

- Opening light for quick ventilation.
- Security for ground floor windows.

Floors

- Commercial machines mounted on concrete floors or plinths if necessary.

Doors

- Wide enough for trolleys if used.
- Door and architrave protection to minimize damage by trolleys.
- Vision panel.

2.3 Interior design

2.3.1 Colour and light

Perception

Older people see the world differently and it follows that the design of spaces for them needs to take account of the perceptual world they inhabit. The kinds of visual problems which will be experienced by some if not all the residents of a care home include:

- restricted vision tending towards blindness: people aged 60 may need three times as much light as people aged 20 to carry out similar visual tasks;
- loss of peripheral vision, or 'tunnel' vision;
- thickening and yellowing of the lens of the eye: the world has a golden glow as in nostalgic advertisements; reds yellows and oranges are more readily distinguished than blues and greens, and it is difficult to distinguish between dark colours; objects against similarly coloured backgrounds may not be distinguished easily, so contrast is important;
- slow and difficult focusing; this can lead to misjudgements of depth and distance;
- disturbing glare; objects cannot be easily seen against bright light; glare can cause older people to stop in their tracks in a state of complete disorientation;
- people with dementia may have the problems listed above exacerbated by cognitive difficulties, e.g. lines on the floor may be seen as steps, or pictures as real objects.

Layout and planning

Orientation

We subconsciously depend on a whole range of perceptual information to tell us where we are. The view ahead is backed up by our peripheral vision, sound, smell, memory and tactile information about the feel of the floor, temperature and air movement. Older people do not get all this information so orientation becomes a much more difficult task.

- The layout of buildings for older people should be clear. Ideally it should be possible to see the day space from the bedroom door.
- There should be as many clues to orientation as possible.
- Colour can be used to differentiate parts of the building.
- Long internal corridors are very confusing, particularly in a big building where they all look the same. Their disadvantages can be mitigated by careful use of colour, windows, automatic hold open devices on the doors, bright lighting of changes in direction and destinations.

Glare

Avoid situations where people will be looking directly at a bright light, for example a long dark corridor with an unshaded window at the end. Shiny reflective surfaces, particularly to floors are not suitable.

Interior design

Lighting

- Generally spaces need to be light and bright without glare.
- Centres of activity like dayrooms should be well lit. Variation in lighting levels between circulation spaces and destinations help people to orientate themselves. There is evidence that older people and especially the mentally frail are attracted to and make for the light.
- Changes in level and direction need to be highlighted.
- Hazards should be lit, preferably at low level.
- Lighting should be designed to flatter residents. Good modelling is desirable.
- Light fittings should be selected to avoid glare.
- Light fittings should be robust and tamper proof, particularly where some residents may be mentally frail.

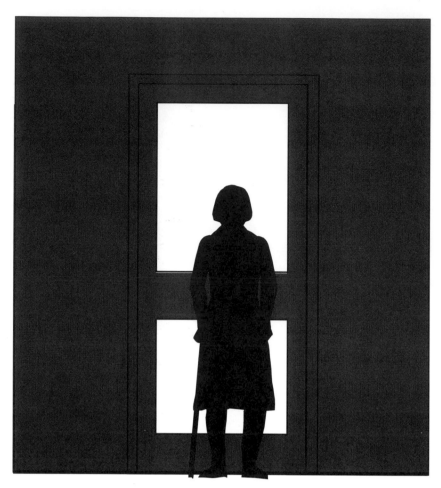

Glare. Daylight and a view out are desirable but glazed doors at the end of dark corridors are a source of glare. Shading devices or additional artificial or day lighting with a sideways component may be needed

Decoration and furniture

- Colour schemes can be helpful in differentiating parts of the building. The choice of colour should be influenced by the problems of perception of blues, greens and dark colours.
- Walls, doors and frames liable to be marked by trolleys and wheelchairs should have guards or be finished with materials which do not show marks.
- Carpets and furnishing fabrics liable to be stained by spills or incontinence should be mottled or patterned. Plain fabrics and carpets show tidemarks after cleaning.

Highlighting

Highlighting of areas or artefacts can be designed into the colour scheme. Contrasting colours will aid identification of the following:

- bedroom doors
- handrails
- toilet doors
- stair nosings
- changes in level or gradient.

Design for dementia

Spaces should be easily recognized for what they are. People with dementia find it easier to know what to do next if they can interpret the space they are in. So it is helpful if bathrooms look like domestic bathrooms (not dentists' consulting rooms). The sight of a recognizable toilet may remind a demented person to use it. Dining rooms with sideboards and tables laid remind people to eat.

- Spaces decorated with familiar looking patterns are an aid to orientation. What looks familiar to older people is the style and decor of their middle age.
- Some fabrics and papers are said to be irritating and distracting, particularly to confused residents. Realistic drawings of objects can be mistaken for the actual thing, and it is frustrating trying to pick an apple from the wallpaper.

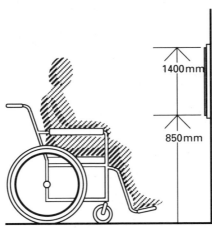

best height of sign for wheelchair user

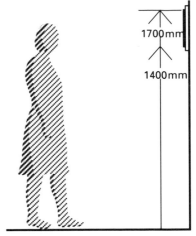

best height of sign for ambulant older person

Sign design

legibility

For easy legibility use
– white letters on dark backgrounds
– bold sans serif typeface
– non-reflective surface
– large letters

- High contrast geometric or striped patterns are not recommended.
- Floor finishes should not have patterns or contrasting colour changes which can be misinterpreted as steps.

Camouflage

Camouflage can be used to deter residents from going into rooms which may be hazardous to them or to conceal scuff marks or stains.

- Doors leading to utility rooms, laundries, lift motor rooms, kitchens, cleaner's stores etc., can be decorated to merge into the background.

Signage

Too many signs give an institutional feel to a building, but undoubtedly they can help people find their way about, and safety signs are essential. The visual clutter can be reduced by co-ordinating the signage at the design stage to avoid a plethora of styles. Fire notices can be co-ordinated with room signs and notice boards provided in key locations like staffrooms and main entrances where there is a need to dispense information.

- Signs should be located within residents' reading range.
- Light letters on a dark background are easiest to read.
- Sans serif typeface is recommended for legibility.
- Signs should be made of a non-reflective material.
- Letters need to be large, minimum size 20 mm.
- Lower case letters are easier to recognize than capitals.
- Use of symbols or logos may be unintelligible to some residents. Old fashioned language may be more appropriate, for example 'ladies' and 'gentlemen' on the toilet doors rather than 'men' and 'women' or pictograms.

2.3.2 Acoustics and sound insulation

Acoustics

All residents are likely to have some hearing loss in the high frequency range.

This means that it is difficult to distinguish consonants and speech thus becomes unintelligible. Loud noises and background noise can still be heard and are irritating as they further interfere with the ability to make out what is being said.

Acoustic design should aim to magnify high frequency sound and minimize background noise.

- Residents need to be near sources of direct sound.
- Reflected sounds should be minimized. Reverberation times need to be short.
- Rooms with hard parallel surfaces of similar sound absorption should be avoided. Irregular shapes produce less echo, alternatively opposed surfaces need to have sound absorbent finishes.
- Columns or pilasters in rooms cast acoustic shadows. Where rooms are used for entertainments or religious services there should be no columns between direct sound sources and residents.
- Background noise level should be kept low. The sources of background noise in care homes are many. Alarm bells, conversations, television and radio, laying and clearing meals, kitchens and laundries, trolleys, toilet flushing, and building maintenance can all impact on the main day areas making communication with some of the residents virtually impossible. It is worth doing a projected background noise audit on the main spaces. Extraneous noises should be eliminated at source if possible or additional absorbent finishes added.

Audio-frequency induction loops

A dramatic improvement in hearing and clarity is possible for people with hearing aids if an induction loop is used. There is a good case for a loop in the main dayroom. The technology is fairly simple and an installation is not particularly expensive, although it must be carried out by a specialist.

An induction loop enables an audio-frequency signal to be transmitted to a hearing aid by means of a magnetic field. A wire loop of insulated cable is mounted at approximately head height around a space. A current flowing through the wire creates a magnetic field which can be picked up by a small coil in a hearing aid. The loop can be connected to a microphone and to television, radio and sound systems. The fluctuating sound signals are transmitted to the hearer via the magnetic field. Most hearing aids are equipped with the coils, including NHS ones. The listener activates the pick up coil by switching the hearing aid to the 'T' position. Listening units with headphones are available for people who do not have hearing aids.

The Royal National Institute for the Deaf publishes a list of installers. Refer to BS 7594 for further information

Telephones

Telephone handsets should be fitted with inductive couplers for use with hearing aids.

Sound insulation

Privacy

Spaces where private conversations need to take place include:

- interview rooms
- manager's or matron's office
- bed-sitting rooms,
- staffroom.

Table 2.1 gives an indication of sound transmittance achieved by different weighted sound reduction indices.

Sound reduction indices of partition systems can be obtained from manufacturers' data but should be used with some caution. In practice small

Table 2.1 Sound reduction targets

Weighted sound reduction index (db)	Acoustic privacy
30	**loud speech can be heard clearly**
35	**loud speech can be distinguished under normal conditions**
40	**loud speech can be heard but not distinguished**
45	**loud speech can be heard faintly but not distinguished**
50+	**loud speech or shouting can be heard with great difficulty**

Reproduced with permission from British Gypsum Ltd. (1991)

holes and gaps left in construction mean that the sound reduction achievable is about 5 dB less than the laboratory rating. Doors in partitions have a further downgrading effect.

Noise control

A combination of absorption and sound insulation is needed to reduce noise levels. Noise sources which cause complaints in care homes are:

- toilets
- kitchens
- laundries
- utility room with automatic sluice
- lifts and lift motor rooms
- footsteps from an upstairs corridor
- trolleys
- laying and clearing tables
- televisions and radios at high volume.

Impact sound

Impact sound is more likely to be a problem between floors than between rooms. A chipboard floor on timber joists with a plasterboard ceiling gives a poor resistance to impact sound (78 dB). In the case of impact sound, lower ratings indicate better performance as opposed to airborne sound ratings where higher numbers indicate sound reduction, i.e. better performance. The Building Regulations require a mean value of 61 dB between floors in dwellings. If impact sound is felt to be a problem it is far easier to take measures to reduce it before the building is built than afterwards.

Building layout implications

Noise control is a consideration when making early planning decisions. For example, distressed residents, especially those with dementia, can be noisy at times. It may take some time for staff to calm an upset person, and in the meantime the noise they make can be painful and disturbing to other residents and visitors.

- Bathing and hair washing lead to trouble quite frequently, and it is preferable to locate these activities away from the public areas.
- Small remote lounges enable a staff member to deal with a distressed person without upsetting others.
- Storage rooms, utility rooms and toilets can be used to isolate noisy rooms from living and bedroom areas.
- External noise sources should be considered.

2.4 Services

This section deals with aspects of services which are specific to the design of care homes rather than services in general.

2.4.1 Heating and ventilation

Room temperatures

Recommended room temperatures are given in Table 2.2.

Table 2.2 Recommended room temperatures

Space	Recommended temperature (°C)
Entrance	23
Bathroom	23
Dayroom	23
Dining room	23
Kitchenette	23
Bedroom	23
Hairdressing	23
Treatment/clinic	23
Nurse station	21
Office	21
Staff room	21
Staff shower	21
Circulation spaces	21
Residents' toilets	21
Kitchen	18
Laundry	18
Utility	18
Stores	18
Staff toilet	18

Surface temperatures

Older people are at greater risk from burning than the general population. The skin becomes more susceptible to burns and reactions are slower. People with dementia are particularly at risk as they may not be able to associate pain with its cause, so they may not move away from a burning surface. There is also the risk that a frail older person may fall against a heat source and be unable to move away. Burns and scalding are in fact the most common cause of accidental death per annum in NHS premises.

All exposed hot pipes and heat sources within reach of residents will need protection. The maximum safe surface temperature is 43°C.

Temperature control

In addition to weather sensors and thermostatic room temperature controls, some consideration may be given to individual temperature controls in bedrooms. One of the most commonly reported causes of frustration reported by residents in care homes is the inability to control their own environment.

Ventilation

Mechanical ventilation is required for kitchens, laundries, toilet and bathroom areas. Good natural ventilation is the minimum requirement for dining areas, residents' bedrooms and day areas.

2.4.2 Electrics

Power supply

Power consumption in care homes is relatively high, particularly where electricity is used for heating. Some upgrading of the main supply will probably be needed in all but the smallest homes; 3-phase supplies will be needed for the following:

- lift
- kitchen
- laundry
- boiler room
- automatic sluice or bed pan washer.

Switches

- Switches intended for use by residents should be within easy reach. Preferred mounting heights are shown in the figure below.
- People should not bend or stretch to reach the switch.
- Switches should have a positive action.
- Consideration should be given to the provision of rocker, push or touch switches for the lights.
- Double sockets should have switches on the outside.
- Dimmer switches may be required in bedrooms.

Lighting

High, glare-free levels of illumination are required. Recommended light levels and limiting glare indices taken from the CIBSE Code for Interior Lighting (1994) can be found in section 2.2. The guide recommends that the levels

Switch and socket fixing heights

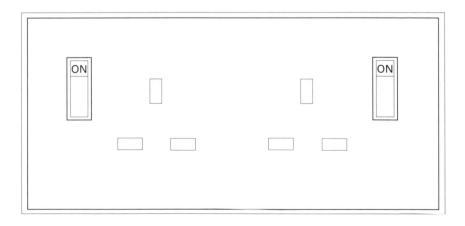

switches and pulls: level with door handle, 900–1050 mm above floor, max 1200 mm above floor
sockets: 700–900 mm above floor

Switches on the outside of sockets are easier for older people to manipulate

shown should be considered as general amenity levels which will need to be substantially increased in hazardous areas such as stairs and kitchenettes. Some Registration Authorities impose standards above the CIBSE levels.

Television

- A television aerial with booster if necessary will be needed.
- Most residents will have their own televisions. Some homes provide video channels to the residents rooms and the dayrooms.

Telephone installation

Individual requirements vary but most homes will need the following provision:

Administration

- Main switch board: manager's office or reception desk
- Extensions to: manager or matron
    nurse stations
    day areas
    kitchen
    laundry.

Monitored line

There should be a separate monitored line to the local Fire Station or line monitoring station.

Residents

Residents should be able to make and receive telephone calls in private. The options are:

- telephone sockets with private line facility in bedrooms; each resident is billed separately;
- payphones (phones on mobile trolleys will be needed for those with restricted mobility; it should be possible to use the phone in private);
- induction loops fitted to residents' telephones.

Lightening conductor

Exposed buildings may require lightening conductors.

2.4.3 Water

Water supply

Infrastructure charges can be calculated on a per capita basis for new or upgraded water supplies and should be ascertained early. They are a major budget item.

Surface temperatures

Hot water temperature

Safe maximum temperature of hot water to resident and visitor areas is 43°C except for bidets, where the maximum is 37–38°C. Thermostatic mixers are required to all hot taps.

Fail-safe devices as specified in BS 1415 part 2 are needed for baths and showers. Hand basins may use single control mechanical mixers starting from cold with a tamper-proof stop to limit full hot water flow. The stop should be set on each device when there is no other hot water demand so the maximum outlet temperature is 40–43°C.

Hot pipe guards

Where hot water pipes are exposed they will need to be guarded if the temperature exceeds 43°C.

Control of Legionella infection

Legionnaires' disease

This has been identified as a major threat to older people and care homes are required to take specific precautions against it. The disease is a form of pneumonia. Those most at risk are people over the age of 50, males, people with a history of respiratory problems and smokers.

Cause	Inhaling an aerosol spray of water infected with the *Legionella* bacteria. Tests have shown that legionellae breed readily in water at a temperature range of around 30–45°C. Water circulation systems have been found to be the cause of all major outbreaks of the diseases. The bacterium is common in water.
Precautions for prevention	• Regular cleaning and purging of the water supply system. • Testing of new installed systems. • Hot water to be circulated at 60°C. Minimum allowable temperature in main circuit is 50°C. • Dead legs to be minimized. The maximum permissible length of dead leg is 5 m. • Unused outlets to be taken out of the system. • Maximum length of pipe with blended water is 2 m. (This means that virtually every hot water outlet needs its own thermostat.)
Further information	The following documents (full details in Further reading) should be consulted: Health and Safety Executive (1991); Department of Health (1991); Brundett (1992).
2.4.4 Emergency power	Care homes are required to make contingency plans for standby heating and lighting in the event of power failure. Power failures can last several days and it should be possible to heat and light by alternative means the parts of the building used by residents. Mobile heating and lighting can be used. The best option is the facility to switch the heating controls and part of the lighting circuit to a standby generator.

2.5 Systems

2.5.1 Security	Care homes are semi-public buildings, as vulnerable as others to threat of theft, vandalism, personal attack or intrusion. Crime prevention considered at the planning stage is cheaper and more effective than adding systems retrospectively. Some homes are located in more vulnerable areas than others, and it is advisable to liaise with the local crime prevention officer at an early stage to assess the level of risk. Each police division has an officer.
Risks	
Burglary	Burglary can be planned or opportunist. Targets are safes, medical supplies and equipment, electrical goods and equipment, televisions, radios, CD players, computers, etc.
Theft in-house	The most commonly reported crime is in-house. This consists of petty theft of kitchen stores, medical and household equipment or theft from residents of small valuables or money.
Vandalism	Casual destruction of property or equipment can be a serious problem in some areas.
Personal attack	The fear of personal attack may be more of a problem than its incidence merits, although there have been attacks on both staff and residents in care homes. Night staff feel particularly vulnerable at the change of shift. Residents in ground-floor rooms may feel at risk.
Confidentiality	Personal records of staff and residents should not be seen by unauthorized people.
Residents' financial affairs	The financial affairs of residents should not be handled by staff or managers of the care home.

Remedies

Visibility

Both inside and outside areas should be designed for good surveillance. Outside spaces, particularly from the car park to the entrance should be well lit. In some circumstances the installation of surveillance systems may be considered.

Entry control

Entry points to the building should be restricted to one or two, which can be supervised. Where there is no receptionist on duty, entryphones may be appropriate. Security of the service or kitchen entrance needs consideration; these doors are sometimes in remote unmonitored parts of the building, and may be left open while deliveries take place.

Secure areas

Some parts of the building will require special security measures. High risk areas like food and drug storage rooms may be better with no windows and specific theft prevention measures may be required by the Registration Authority.

Residents' rooms

Rooms should be lockable. Where there is a risk of residents locking themselves accidentally in their rooms locks can be fitted to the outside of the door only. At least each resident should have a lockable drawer or cupboard for small valuables.

Windows and doors

Ground-floor windows and doors should be secure.

2.5.2 Fire prevention

Design guidance

Residential and Nursing Homes for older people are in purpose group 2(a) Residential (Institutional). The usual assumption that the building should be designed for unaided evacuation of all occupants cannot apply where at least some will be bedridden or have very limited mobility. The principle of progressive horizontal evacuation of the occupants into adjoining compartments is usually adopted. Design guidance is available in the following documents: Department of Health (1987; 1989); Home Office (1982; 1983); Building Regulations (1991) and local authority or health authority registration requirements. Registration authorities must ensure that buildings are in accordance with one of the standard guidelines and the Building Regulations. There may be additional local requirements; for example many authorities insist on the provision of a monitored line to the Fire Brigade or to a monitoring station.

Fire and older people

Many older people fear fire and it is often mentioned as a major concern by those moving in to residential care. In general residents like to feel they are in a safe building and do not object to overt fire precautions. There are times when there is conflict between the needs of older people and the demands of fire safety; what may be satisfactory in buildings for the general population will not be adequate. The areas needing special consideration are discussed below.

Self-closing devices

Most self-closing devices present an impassable barrier to many of the people likely to be resident in a care home, except rising butt hinges but these do not give adequate fire protection. The installation of automatic door releases connected to the fire alarm system is the best solution to this problem. Hold open devices are appropriate for doors across corridors and free swing devices for room doors. These devices are not allowed where the door leads to an escape stair and it is best if the circulation routes in daily use by residents do not cross stair enclosures.

Alarms

Consideration should be given to the installation of visual as well as audio alarms for the benefit of the deaf.

| Emergency lighting | Emergency lighting should be designed for people with poor sight. |

| Furnishing materials | Furniture and fabrics should be either inherently flame retardant or treated with flame retardant. Where residents are encouraged to bring their own furniture into the home it may not comply with the British Standard ignitability tests. The issue will need to be discussed in detail with the Registration Authority and the Fire Prevention Officer; it may be appropriate to treat upholstery fabrics with a durable flame retardant or to install additional smoke detectors. |

| Fire escape doors | In homes for the mentally infirm there may be a requirement to constrain access to the outside to prevent the residents from wandering off. Various design solutions are adopted depending on the degree of constraint deemed appropriate. Low key distraction techniques are best and should be adopted wherever possible. Locking people in will be a cause of frustration to them. This option should only be adopted where there is no better alternative and the risks justify the restriction. |

Some of the methods used are:

- Mirrors. A mirror fixed to an external door is an effective way of stopping confused people. They become distracted by their own reflection and may lose track of the intention of wandering outside.
- Secure outside enclosed spaces. It does not matter very much if a demented resident wanders into a safe enclosed outside space. The fire door can have an alarm linked to the nurse call system so the staff know that someone has got out.
- Double door handles. Two door handles can be fitted, one at high level. This may be sufficiently confusing to some (but not all) demented residents to deter them. Any system which restricts free egress from fire doors must be agreed with the Fire Authority.
- Automatic door releases. Door releases connected to the fire alarm system keep fire doors locked except in an emergency. Access for staff may be by means of switches or keys located at high level. Such a system should be discussed with and approved by the Fire Authority.

2.5.3 Nurse call

| Types of installation | - Wired system to central control panel. Calls are recorded on the central control panel. Additional slave panels can be fitted around the building. Radio paging of staff or speech intercom can be included. When a call is made an alarm sounds. Staff go to the nearest panel to locate the call.
- Radio system to central control panel. This is similar to the wired system operationally. Radio paging of staff or speech intercom can be included. Installation is simpler as there is no wiring. A transmitter and receiver are fitted and additional aerials and boosters as required.
- Follow the light wired system. The building is divided into four or five zones. When a call is made an alarm sounds. A light comes on outside the room door and simultaneously flashing light panels in prominent positions around the building indicate the call zone. Staff go to the zone to locate the call. This system uses less wiring as there is no need for each call point to connect to a central panel. |

| Location of call points | Positions of call points are shown in the figure overleaf.

The areas of the building which need alarm call points are indicated in Table 2.3. |

| Linked communications | The nurse call system can be extended to include other communications as shown in Table 2.4. |

Nurse call point

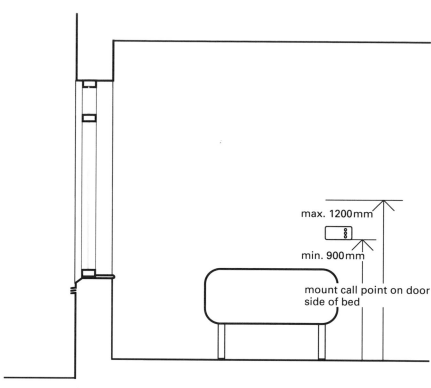

max. 1200mm

min. 900mm

mount call point on door
side of bed

wall-mounted nurse call point

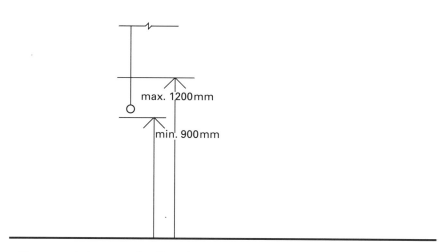

max. 1200mm

min. 900mm

ceiling-mounted nurse call pull cord

System controls

Staff need to be able to monitor the nurse call system from various locations as indicated in Table 2.5.

System monitoring

Central control panel systems can be logged. Print-outs can record time of calls, response time and room checks where no call is made.

Alarm systems for confused residents

Specialist homes for very frail or confused older people may have different needs. Where residents are not capable of using the nurse call system, nurse-to-nurse communication only is required. In general the call points should not be easily accessible to residents. There may also be a need for non-intrusive monitoring of residents by staff so that, for example, anybody falling out of bed or wandering off the site does not go unnoticed.

Call points

The call points in Table 2.6 are for the use of staff.

Linked communications

The nurse call system can be extended to include other communications as shown in Table 2.7.

Table 2.3 Call point locations

Space	Position	Call unit	Staff facility
Bedroom	Bedhead	Wall-mounted push button with extension lead (long enough to reach seats) and reassurance light	Reset, call assistance, call emergency
Toilet	Within reach of of toilet	Red pull cord with reassurance light	Wall-mounted reset, call assistance, call emergency
Bath or shower	Within reach of bath or shower and toilet	Red pull cord with reassurance light	Wall-mounted reset, call assistance, call emergency
Dayrooms	Within reach and in sight of staff and residents; avoid furniture; avoid confusion with light switch	Wall-mounted push button with extension lead (long enough to reach seats) and reassurance light	Reset, call assistance, call emergency
Dining	Within reach and in sight of staff and residents; avoid furniture; avoid confusion with light switch	Wall-mounted push button with reassurance light	Reset, call assistance, call emergency
Circulation	Within reach of staff	Wall-mounted push button	Reset, call assistance, call emergency

Table 2.4 Communications linked to nurse call system

Origin	Position	Call unit	Staff facility
Front door bell	Front door	Door bell; entryphone	Reset, call assistance, call emergency
Drug store	Door to store or cupboard	Magnetic microswitch indicates when door is opened; red warning light over door	Reset, call assistance, call emergency
Night time telephone call	Main switch board	Telephone bell	Telephone extension

Table 2.5 Nurse call system controls

Space	Central control panel system	Follow light system
Nurse station	Main control panel or slave panel	Zone indicator panel
Manager's office	Main control panel or slave panel	
Matron's office	Main control panel or slave panel	
Staff room	Slave panel	Zone indicator panel
Each floor or wing	Slave panel	Zone indicator panel
Point of origin of call	Reset, call assistance, call emergency	Over door light, reset, call assistance, call emergency
All areas of building	Alarm sounders, three tones, volume increase if required, mutable at night	Alarm sounders, three tones, volume increase if required, mutable at night

Table 2.6 Call point locations for confused residents

Space	Position	Call unit	Staff facility
Bedroom	Bedhead or room door	Wall-mounted push button out of reach of resident	Reset, call assistance, call emergency
Toilet	Room entry	Wall-mounted push button out of reach of resident	Reset, call assistance, call emergency
Bath or shower	Within reach of bath or shower and toilet	Wall-mounted push button out of reach of resident	Reset, call assistance, call emergency
Dayrooms	Within reach and in sight of staff; avoid furniture; avoid confusion with light switch	Wall-mounted push button out of reach of resident	Reset, call assistance, call emergency
Dining	Within reach and in sight of staff; avoid furniture; avoid confusion with light switch	Wall-mounted push button out of reach of resident	Reset, call assistance, call emergency
Circulation	Within reach of staff	Wall-mounted push button	Reset, call assistance, call emergency

Table 2.7 Communication links to nurse call; confused residents

Origin	Position	Call unit	Staff facility
Fire escape door	Door frame	Magnetic microswitch indicates when door is opened	Reset, call assistance, call emergency
Bedhead	Bed	Movement sensor, pressure pad, infrared curtain	Reset, call assistance, call emergency

2.6 Site

2.6.1 Location and site selection

Neighbourhood

Homes are best located within the communities from which they obtain their clientele, so the residents know the area and their friends and neighbours (who are also likely to be old) can visit.

Care staff often work part time and on shifts and prefer to work near home. Most staff will be recruited from the immediate neighbourhood. An established residential area with a population which includes older people and families with older children, preferably without other employment options available is ideal.

Local facilities

Access to local facilities is required. Centres need to be very near to be of benefit to residents. Only about 50% of residents are likely to go out on their own, and those who do are unlikely to travel more than 100–200 m, or less in a hilly area. The quality of the paving, street lighting, pedestrian crossings and the availability of seating will affect the residents' ability to go out. Facilities desirable within walking distance are shops, post office, health centre, hairdressers, dentist and pub. An idealized location is shown in the drawing opposite.

Building design guide

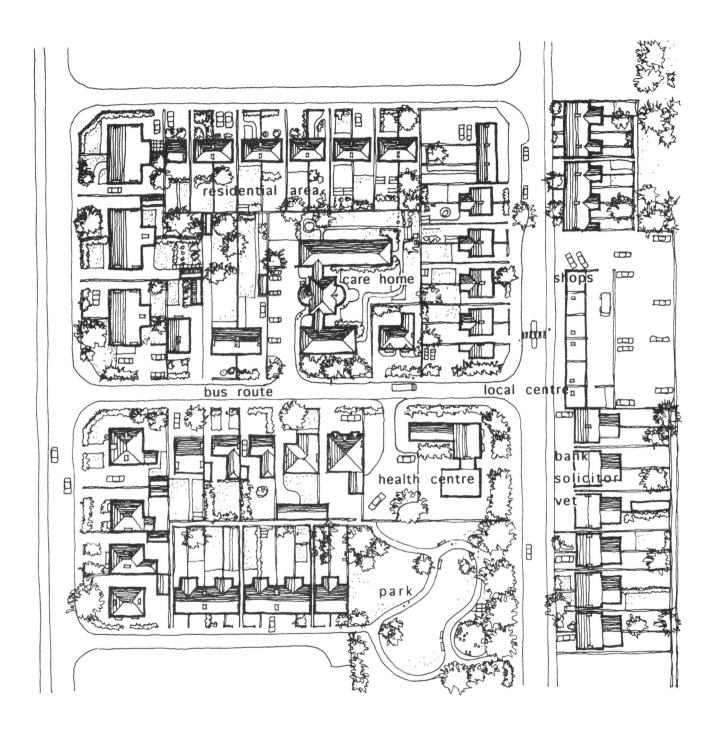

residential area

care home

shops

bus route

local centre

health centre

bank

solicitor

vet

park

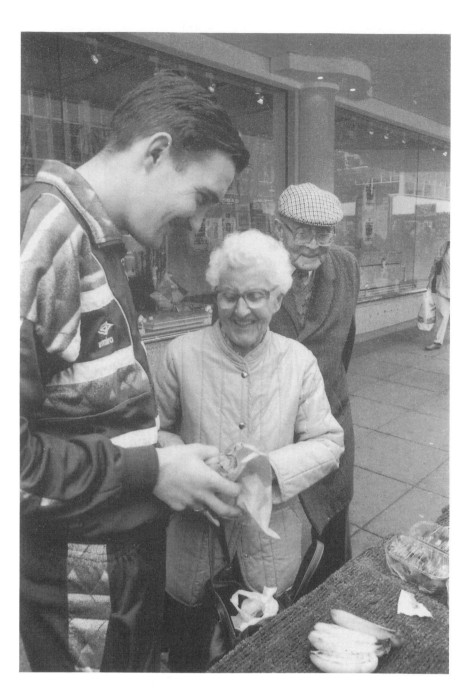

Visits to churches, cinemas, clubs and community centres are likely to be made by car or taxi. These amenities should not be more than half a kilometre away.

Transport links

Older people are dependant on public transport. Homes should be on bus routes, and bus stops need to be very near to be of use to residents or their visitors. Ideally the bus stop should be within 50 m of the front door connected to it by a direct path, and should be provided with shelter and a seat. It is likely that this will fall inside the visibility splay required by the Highway Authority (see section 2.6.2. below) and a certain amount of negotiation will be needed with the Highways Authority and the bus service provider to get the bus stop in the right place.

Road access

Homes should be served by adopted roads of a standard suitable for fire appliances, refuse vehicles and service vehicles.

Community links

Day centres and sheltered housing for older people living in the community can be sited adjacent to care homes. The advantage of this arrangement is

Day areas need views of local
activities

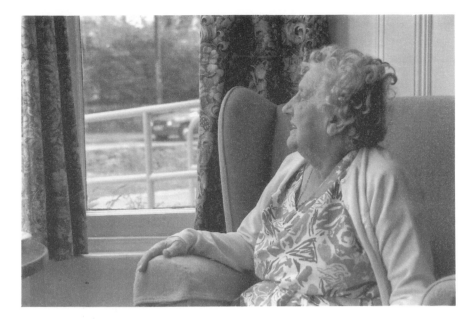

that people become familiar with the home before moving in, but it is important that such facilities do not intrude on the privacy of the residents in the care home.

Activity

Since 50% of the residents are unlikely to go out, homes should be sited to take advantage of any activity on or off the site. Regular movements of schoolchildren, building workers or delivery vehicles are interesting to watch.

A building which generates a lot of activity such as a fire station makes an ideal neighbour.

Security

Buildings should be sited in a safe area. Special precautions to combat vandalism or theft may be appropriate.

Competition

Homes which are too close to each other will inevitably compete for residents and staff.

Neighbours

Although care homes are in fact unobtrusive neighbours there are likely to be objections to planning applications. Objections are likely to be on the grounds of commercialization of a residential area and overlooking. Care homes are not generally held in high regard. Planning restrictions to prevent overlooking are illustrated in the diagram overleaf.

Cost

The direct relationship between site cost and residents' fees leads to intensive site development. Constraints are the size of home the authority will register, distance to adjacent buildings, storey height, car parking and access requirements. There is no necessity for large gardens; small linked sheltered spaces around the site are more appropriate for older people.

2.6.2 Vehicle and pedestrian access

Vehicle entrance

The requirements of Highway Authorities differ in detail and should be checked early for each development. The principal considerations are listed below.

- The access must be a safe distance from the nearest road junction. Acceptable spacing between centres of junctions on the same side can be 44–55 m or greater on fast roads. Opposite side junction spacing is around half the same side spacing, as illustrated below.
- Access drives should be at right angles to the road at the entry point.
- A car waiting to enter the highway should have unobstructed visibility in both

Typical planning restrictions on
distance between buildings
(note: Planning Authorities vary in
their requirements)

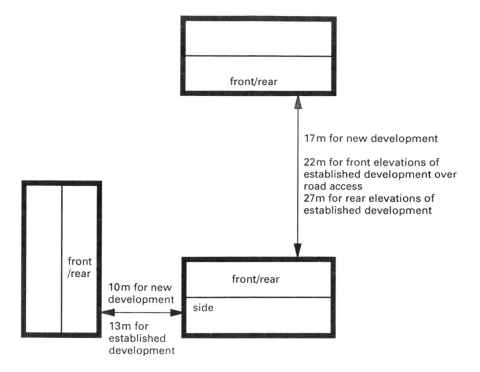

front/rear

17m for new development

22m for front elevations of
established development over
road access
27m for rear elevations of
established development

front
/rear

front/rear

side

10m for new
development

13m for
established
development

single storey

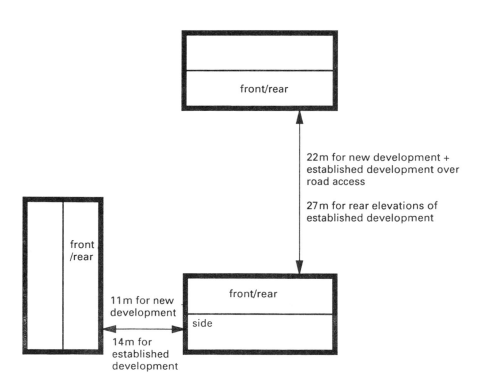

front/rear

22m for new development +
established development over
road access

27m for rear elevations of
established development

front
/rear

front/rear

side

11m for new
development

14m for
established
development

2 storey + 2 storey and single storey

Building design guide

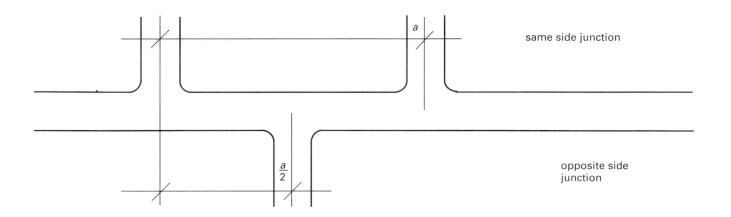

same side junction

opposite side
junction

Distance between access drive and road junction.
Dimension at *a* varies according to area and road speed. Typical values of *a* are 44–55m.

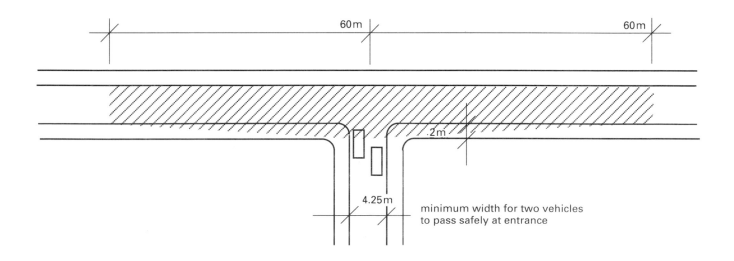

minimum width for two vehicles
to pass safely at entrance

Typical visibility splay for junction with 30 mph road. Faster roads need longer splays.

Site

directions from the driver's eye line. The dimensions of the visibility splay are dependant on the design speed of the road. The drawing on p. 95 shows a typical visibility splay.

- There should be enough width for two vehicles to pass at the point of entry to the highway to avoid obstructing the traffic. Minimum width for two vehicles is 4.25 m.
- Gates are not very practical for care homes. If required they need to be set a minimum of 5 m back from the back of the footway.
- Maximum permitted gradient of access drive is 1:10. Preferred maximum is 1:20.
- Access will be required for fire appliances (see Building Regulations)
- Refuse collection method will need to be agreed with the Local Authority or contractor. There is likely to be a separate collection of clinical waste. BS 5906: 1980 sets out a maximum recommended carry distance for refuse collection of 25 m.

Pedestrian access

- Pedestrians on the footway need a 2 m × 2 m visibility splay so that they can see cars coming to the end of the access drive.
- Minimum path width for one wheelchair is 1200 mm. Preferred width is 1350 mm. Minimum width for two wheelchairs to pass is 1800 mm. Preferred width is 2000 mm.
- Access should be as level as possible. Any gradient steeper than 1:30 will be tiring to an older person dependant on walking aids. Rest areas with seats should be provided at frequent intervals. Seats near the main entrance are popular with older residents who like a good look at who is coming and going.
- Ramps where provided must comply with Building Regulations. Where ramps of 1:20 or steeper are provided steps will be needed as well for semi-ambulant older people who find the ramps too steep.

Car parking

- Minimum car parking bay size is 2.4 m × 5 m.
- Some spaces will be required for wheelchair access. The drawing below shows a wheelchair access shared between two parking bays.
- An ambulance and mini-bus bay may be required by the main entrance.
- One or two parking spaces with wheelchair access should be provided very near the entrance. A covered walkway between the pick-up points and the building is desirable.
- There is a wide variation between parking standards stipulated by different authorities. The least onerous is:

    2 spaces for visitors and staff

    plus 1 space for every 4 bed spaces

    plus an additional space for every resident staff bed space.

    Standards much higher than this are imposed elsewhere, particularly in urban areas, where the rule may be:

Parking bays for wheelchair users

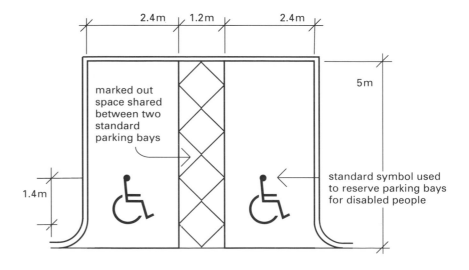

marked out space shared between two standard parking bays

standard symbol used to reserve parking bays for disabled people

Building design guide

1 space for each staff member
plus 1.5 spaces for residential staff and their visitors
plus 1 space for every 3 bed spaces
plus an ambulance bay and parking for the disabled by the entrance
plus a service yard of at least 50 m^2 with turning head.
A reduction in the number of spaces may be negotiated where long-term residents are housed.

2.6.3 Service yards

Waste bin sizes

- A bin storage area will be needed for general and clinical waste. General waste is stored in wheeled bins. Standard 660 litre and 1100 litre bins are illustrated in the diagram below.

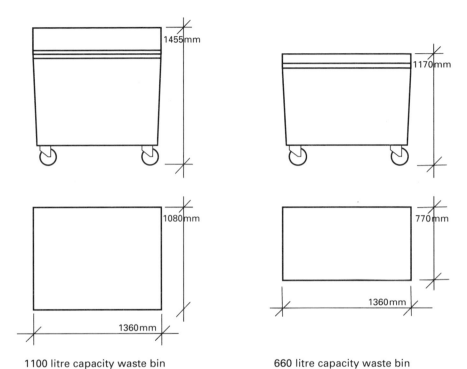

1100 litre capacity waste bin   660 litre capacity waste bin

Bin storage areas need to be convenient for the kitchen but screened and sited away from kitchen windows. The bin store area will need regular washing down; a yard gully and hose point are required.

- Access is required for kitchen deliveries and laundry deliveries where laundry is not done on the premises. Holding areas for soiled linen should be remote from food delivery areas.
- Service vehicles should be able to turn within the site.

2.6.4 Gardens

Layout

Older people benefit even more than the rest of the population from regular fresh air and exercise, yet the gardens of most care homes are chronically underused. Partly this can be explained by the staff failing to make the effort to encourage people outside but often the problem lies in the detailed design of the exterior; the residents just do not find that outside spaces are tailored to their needs. An elderly person on the wrong side of a door which is too heavy to open when an urgent trip to the toilet is needed is put off going outside again.

The design of outside spaces should take into account the lessening abilities of older people.

Mobility

- Paths should be level or laid with gradients less than 1:30 where possible. Frequent resting places with seating are desirable.

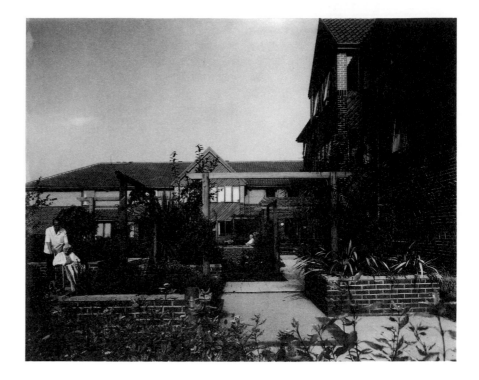

A garden with raised beds and water features. Scented and tactile plants are used for the benefit of people with visual impairments. Churchfield Christian Nursing Home, Architects Design and Build Services Ltd, 1988–1989

- Low obstacles, particularly at ground level, should be avoided. Thresholds and path edgings adjacent to lawns should be flush; there should be no small holes or changes in level which could catch walking sticks or frames.
- Paths need to be wide enough for wheelchairs to pass (1.65 m minimum, 1.8 m preferred).
- Surface finishes should be non-slip and semi-porous (icy surfaces are greatly feared by the old). Gravel or loose surface finishes are inappropriate. Gully gratings are best avoided where older people are likely to walk with walking aids, or, if essential, they need to be firmly fixed with small drainage holes.
- Handrails are as essential outside as inside.
- Good access to toilets from sitting areas is needed.
- The areas and routes nearest the building should be designed for the least mobile. These can link up with longer more challenging walks for the active.
- There will always be some residents who are unable to go out. Bedroom and dayroom windows can be the only link with the outside world, and views from them should be attractive and interesting.

Eyesight

- Good lighting particularly at ground level is important.
- Path edges and step nosings should be clearly identified.
- Colours in the red/orange/yellow sector of the spectrum are more easily seen than blues and greens.
- Signs need to be clear and legible.
- Failing eyesight and hearing mean that orientation becomes more difficult as people age; there are less clues. The best garden layouts are clear and unambiguous. Routes radiating from a recognizable central place or linear paths marked by pauses with distinctive features help people to locate themselves.

Hearing

- Seats arranged close to each other help people to converse.
- Background noise sources can be reduced by screen walls or planting.

Dexterity

- Doors should be very easily opened from both sides.

Thermal comfort

- Control of the micro-climate is important. Older people are susceptible to cold. The ideal garden faces south-west towards the afternoon sun, half enclosed by building with wind break planting at the site perimeter. Sitting areas need to be draught and rain proof.

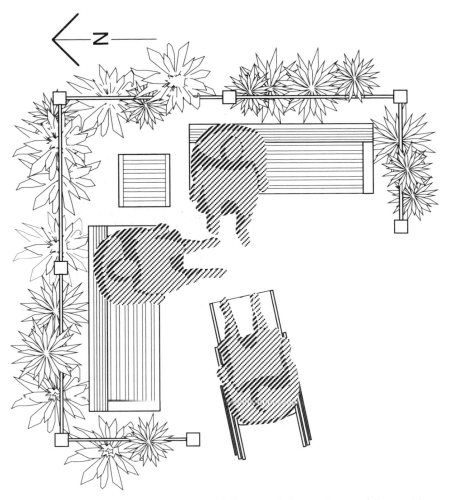

User requirements

These vary according to the type and degree of dependency of the residents. Specialist homes for people with dementia have different needs from homes for the very frail. People with dementia may be physically fit and active and the provision of hands-on gardening opportunities and reasonably challenging walking routes has therapeutic value.

- A patio and seating area linked closely to the dayrooms will be used for sitting, conversation, smoking, barbecues and picnics.
- A wandering route around the garden to include long or shorter routes should be possible. The route should not be boring but marked by interesting diversions: sitting spaces, rose gardens, safe water features, bird tables or animal pens, sensory gardens. Wandering routes are of particular importance to people with dementia.
- For the life-time gardener there is nothing quite like the feel of compost in a pot. The provision of potting sheds, greenhouses, garden plots, raised beds, personal window boxes gives residents scope for gardening. These should be sited with regard to orientation and shading and away from the public gaze.
- Semi-private spaces for families and visitors should be provided.
- Objects of attraction for children and young people make visiting more of a pleasure. These can range from a swing to a swimming pool.
- A securely fenced garden is normally required to prevent people with dementia from wandering off the site and getting lost.
- Seats at the front of the building are always popular.
- Storage for garden maintenance tools and lawn mowers should be provided.

Planting

The gardens should be planted for year-round colour, texture and low maintenance. Planting should not, however, be uniform and dull, a tasteful unchanging background. Spring bulbs, summer flowers, autumn colour and winter texture enable residents to keep in touch with passing seasons within

Top. Raised bed

Middle. Raised bed

Bottom. Adjustable height
gardening tray for wheelchair users

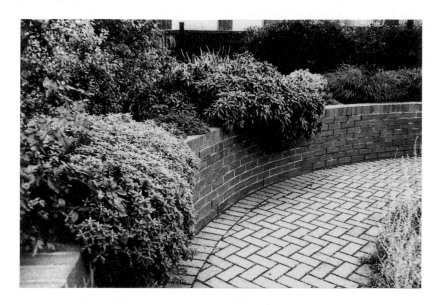

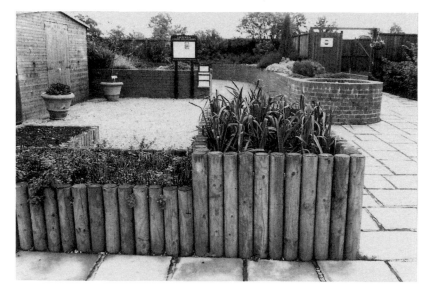

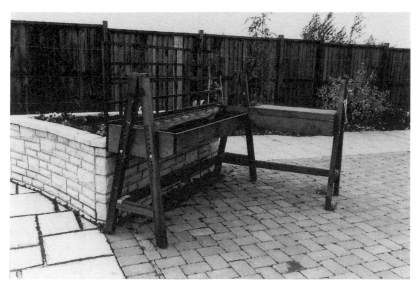

their inevitably restricted horizons. Native plants and fruits attract wildlife including birds; bird tables can be sited outside resident's windows. The progress of fruit and vegetables through the growing season is of interest to anyone who has enjoyed gardening.

Planting at high level can be enjoyed by people in wheelchairs. Illustrated opposite are raised beds at Ryton Gardens. The plants are chosen for fragrance and texture so that they can be enjoyed by people with poor eyesight.

- Plants to avoid include poisonous and harmful plants and those with sharp thorns or cutting edges. It is common for people with dementia to pick and eat both garden and indoor plants. A list of poisonous and harmful plants published by The Horticultural Trades Association appears in Technical Supplement 3.

Red, orange, yellow and white flowers will have more impact than blues and purples.

Lighting

- Security lighting is required at the entrance and car parks to reduce the risk of theft, for the safety of night staff changing shifts and around the site to deter thieves and vandals. Depending on the degree of risk, security lighting can be backed up by video cameras.
- Amenity lighting may be required at the site entrance and signboard. It can also be used to highlight the patio and gardens at night.
- Safety lighting will be required for footpaths, ramps and steps. It is best sited at low level.
- Lighting design needs early consideration, particularly if extensive cabling is required. Cable routes and depths need to be planned with a view to economy, maintenance and safety. Lights fixed to the building are the cheapest option.

Detail design

Seating

- Seats need to be warm, protected from wind and rain in a sunny position.
- Seats at right angles make it easier for people to hear each other.
- There should be room for a wheelchair user to join a seated group.
- Seats alongside a path should not obstruct the route. There should not be a change in level or surface finish under the seat.
- Concrete or metal seats are cold to the touch. Wood, plastic or cushions are better. Drainage holes or slats in the seat prevent water collecting.
- Seats must be strong and stable. Old people tend to lower themselves down using the arm rests and it is important that the seat does not slip backwards.
- A kick space of at least 75 mm behind the front edge of the chair seat will be needed for people to lower themselves into the seat.

Seating design parameters

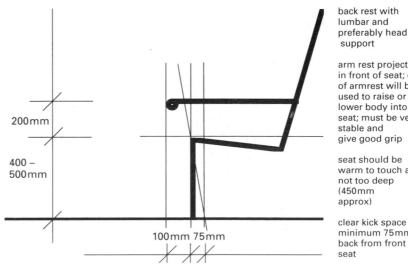

200mm

400 –
500mm

100mm 75mm

back rest with lumbar and preferably head support

arm rest projecting in front of seat; end of armrest will be used to raise or lower body into seat; must be very stable and give good grip

seat should be warm to touch and not too deep (450mm approx)

clear kick space minimum 75mm back from front of seat

Table heights and thigh clearances.
Avoid bars at low level. Table top
should have rounded corners and
edges

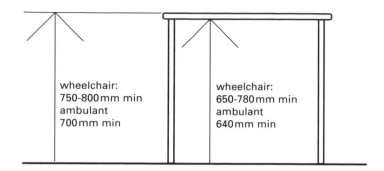

wheelchair:
750-800mm min
ambulant
700mm min

wheelchair:
650-780mm min
ambulant
640mm min

- Good back and if possible head support is needed.
- Tables associated with sitting areas should be suitable for wheelchairs.

Handrails

- Handrails are required at the entrances to the building to enable the least mobile to gain access to the dropping-off points by the front door and the patio areas associated with the dayrooms.
- Handrails are required at ramps and changes in level, and for guarding against hazards.
- The more extensive the handrail provision the more accessible the garden will be to the residents.

Hands-on planting

The level of provision depends on the category of residents. Some form of gardening may be appropriate for almost everyone, but the less mobile will need working areas very close to the day rooms.

- Raised planting beds are good in that the plants in them are easier for older people to appreciate than those at ground level, and the bed walls provide good mobility aids. They are rather awkward to work for those in wheelchairs because they have to sit sideways on. This can be partly overcome by the provision of knee holes, but at the expense of a decent depth of soil which may lead to disappointing harvests.
- Containers, plant pots and window boxes can be planted up while people are sitting at a table.
- Allotment plots for the more active should not be too large. They should be in good sunlight and reasonably secluded from curious and critical eyes. The gardens will fail unless there is a good depth (400–600 mm) of well fertilized and dug soil.
- Greenhouses are best sited in full sun orientated east-west. The door width will need to be a minimum 800 mm wide to accommodate wheelchairs. Water and electricity supplies may be required.
- Potting sheds should be close to the working areas. A screened area for garden waste and compost heaps will be needed.

Grounds maintenance

- Separate storage space should be provided for lawn mower, maintenance tools and equipment, paint and other sundries. The store should be secure. At least some of the stored items are likely to be a fire risk.

3 Management of the building process

3.1 Statutory approvals and inspections

3.1.1 Registration

Homes for four or more older people must be registered and regularly inspected under the Registered Homes Act 1984. There is a simplified procedure for registering homes for three people or less under the Registered Homes (Amendment) Act 1991.

Health Authorities register and inspect nursing homes which are for people who need regular nursing care. Nursing homes must have a qualified nurse on duty at all times. Homes for people who can no longer manage to live in the community but do not need regular nursing care are called rest or retirement or residential homes and must be registered with and inspected by the Local Authority Social Services Department. The authorities appoint Registration Officers who are responsible for the registration and inspection of homes subject to committee approval. The Registration Officer may be supported by technical staff.

Registration guidelines

Each authority has a set of registration guidelines. The requirements are similar but by no means identical, and they are regularly updated. Authorities charge for registration guideline packs; they cost around £100 a set. All aspects of home running are covered from staffing ratios and drugs control to space standards and services. It is essential to work to an up-to-date set of guidelines and to check that they will not be superseded by the time the building is registered. Registration can only take place when the building is ready to admit residents and a prior approval of a plan in principle does not guarantee registration if the requirements have changed. Registration Officers are available for consultation and will usually comment in writing on proposals for new buildings but their recommendations are subject to committee approval. It is not unknown for additional conservatories to be built on at the last minute to accommodate an increase in the space standards for dayrooms.

Registration requirements are based on national guidelines. Broadly the same areas are covered but the detail varies considerably; some authorities for instance ask for nearly twice as much dayroom space as others.

Registration is granted to an individual who is either the owner or the manager responsible for providing the service. This must be a named individual rather than a partnership or association. Where a manager is appointed who is responsible for running the home, that person must also be registered.

The guidelines are not written exclusively for building designers and specifiers. They need to be read carefully to pick up all the references to building requirements. There may be a section dealing with accommodation, but there are likely to be essential parts of the building brief in other parts of the document; for instance, within the guidelines on drug administration there may be a reference to the need to bolt the drugs trolley to a masonry wall; this is the sort of problem that can cause trouble in a timber-framed building if not picked up at an early stage.

Requirements	The requirements vary from authority to authority. Those aspects which affect the building may include some or all of the following points.
Location	• Preferred location is within residential areas and with good public transport links. • Access to local shops, churches and community buildings is desirable.
Building size	Many authorities prefer to limit the size of homes to 40 residents although there is pressure from providers to increase this number.

Accommodation schedule

Space standards	• minimum sizes for bedrooms • ratio of single to double rooms • dayroom area per resident • dining area per resident • minimum sizes for bathrooms and toilets • minimum corridor widths.
Sanitary facilities	Minimum numbers of sanitary facilities per resident are always specified. Their location in terms of walking distance from dayrooms and bedrooms may be stipulated. Some authorities impose minimum room sizes and layouts, and there may be requirements for equipment such as mechanical sluices or baths with lifting devices and non-slip bases. Areas covered by regulation include: • bathrooms and shower rooms • toilets • washbasins for residents • staff hand washing and drying facilities (staff should never have to use residents' soap and towels) • sluicing facilities.
Ancillary accommodation	Certain ancillary spaces are mandatory: • staff room • office, or space for keeping records secure • private interview room • staff changing room • separate staff toilets • visitors toilet • separate toilet for the exclusive use of kitchen staff.

Access and mobility

Lifts	Lifts are required for multi-storey buildings. Lift size, installation, commissioning and inspection requirements are usually specified.
Access	• provision and specification of ramps • handrails, grab rails and support rails required along corridors, in lifts, in bathrooms and toilets • corridor width to allow wheelchairs to pass • door width.

Lifting equipment	Mechanical lifting equipment may be required for bathing and lifting residents who fall.

Interior design

Furniture	Minimum bedroom and dayroom provision is required.
Finishes	Floor finishes are most likely to be specified as follows:

- carpet to be washable
- non-slip sealed floors in wet areas
- matwells or entrance matting.

Fittings	

- ironmongery performance specifications may be included, e.g. window opening restraints, bathroom and bedroom locks with emergency access from the outside.
- on sanitary fittings lever handle taps may be specified.

Security	Standards of security will be laid down for some areas such as:

- rooms where drugs are stored; bolting and chaining of drug trolleys, warning lights and door locks
- door and window security
- records storage.

Environment

Heating	The requirements include minimum temperatures, maximum surface temperatures, guarding of heating appliances, provision of back-up heating in the event of power failure.
Ventilation	Ventilation requirements include:

- dayrooms
- bedrooms
- lift motor rooms and the top of lift shafts
- kitchens (provision of fly screens for opening windows in food preparation rooms, ventilation of food stores)
- laundries, drying machines and linen stores.

Lighting	Minimum lighting levels, emergency lighting, location and type of light fittings in bedrooms and dayrooms and corridors.
Fire precautions	Fire precautions standards. There may be specific requirements such as the provision of a monitored telephone line linked to the fire alarm.
Services and systems	Commissioning and regular inspection requirements for all service and systems installations.
Emergency call system	Installation and minimum provision.
Electrical installation	Arrangements for alternative systems in the event of power failure.
Telephone	

- Separate telephones are required for residents' use and administration.
- Public phone must be provided.
- Monitored telephone link to the fire service must be installed.

Water supply	Installation, commissioning and maintenance standards are usually specified. Standards include:

- water temperature range

	• guarding of hot water pipes • storage of water • precautions against Legionnaire's disease in water storage systems • provision of potable water.
Waste disposal	Special arrangements for soiled and clinical waste and sharps disposal.
Home management	Registration guidelines are addressed to home managers, and much of their content is concerned with management standards. The issues covered are listed below.
Resident care	• admission procedures • contract of care • privacy and personal autonomy • financial regulations • health care including terminal care • administration, record keeping • food • community links.
Client group	• specific needs of older people
Staff	• supervision, staff ratios and minimum cover • staff selection • qualifications and training • selection and training of ancillary staff • specialist staff or use of community-based professionals • staff welfare, health and safety.
Statutory requirements	Care homes must comply with current legislation. The registration guidelines refer to relevant Acts of Parliament and Statutory Instruments listed here: • *Registered Homes Act 1984.* • *Draft guide to fire precautions in existing residential care premises*, Home Office 1983. • *Firecode*. Department of Health guidance on fire precautions in health care buildings for use in new NHS buildings. May be used for residential homes. • Home Office *Draft Guide to Fire Precautions in Hospitals for use in existing NHS buildings.* • *Building Regulations 1991* and amendments. • *Town and Country Planning Act 1971.* • *Race Relations Act 1976 (Sections 20 and 22(2)(b))* and *Racial discrimination: a guide to the Race Relations Act 1975.* • *Sex Discrimination Act 1975.* • *Health and Safety at Work Act 1974.* • *Food Safety Act 1990.* • *Food Hygiene (General) Regulations 1970.*
Recommended standards	Guidelines also refer to accepted national standards where possible. They may also require compliance with local bylaws. See also Further reading. Specific reference is commonly made to: • Institute of Electrical Engineers *Guidance for electrical installations.* • *Code for Interior Lighting*. Chartered Institute of Building Services Engineers. • *Water supply bylaws guide*. Water Research Centre. • *Water fittings and materials directory*. Unwin Brothers Ltd, Old Woking, Surrey GU22 9LH. • *The Control of Legionellae in health care premises – a Code of Practice, with amendments 1 and 2.* Department of Health.

- *Approved Code of Practice – The prevention or control of legionellosis (including Legionnaire's disease)*. Health and Safety Executive.
- British Standards.

3.1.2 Approvals and inspections

The registering authority needs documentary evidence that the building has been inspected and approved by other agencies before the home can be registered.

Planning Approval

Copy of Planning Approval and written confirmation by the Planning Officer of compliance with any conditions.

Building Regulations

Copy of Building Regulations Approval and Building Inspector's certificate of completion.

Fire Prevention

Inspection and formal approval of the fire precautions by the Fire Prevention Officer. Fire-retardant certificates in respect of furnishing fabrics.

Environmental Health

Inspection and formal approval.

Health Authority

Confirmation that pharmaceutics storage is satisfactory.

Most registration authorities will require additional certification at registration. This may include the following:

Services and systems

Electric installation

The electrical contractor to provide:

- electrical test notice, completion certificate and electric wiring certificate renewable every 5 years;
- certification of nurse call system;
- certification of fire detection and fire alarm systems.

Gas installation

The system installer to provide:

- installation certificate;
- annual servicing agreement for boiler plant and gas services.

Water installation

The mechanical services contractor to provide:

- certification by Water Inspector that the water installation complies with the bylaws;
- certification that the heating and water installations conform with requirements for prevention of Legionnaire's disease and temperature controls.

Lift and stairlift

Certificates needed:

- test certificate and commissioning report;
- certificate of insurance.

Mechanical lifting devices

Certificates of insurance are needed.

Emergency power

Arrangements for providing temporary heating and lighting in the event of power failure.

3.2 The building process

The production of a care home is a time- and cost-sensitive operation. Building income is reasonably foreseeable, and may even be guaranteed by, for example, Health Authorities, in exchange for private finance, design and construction. The need to limit and predict time and cost of construction accurately has led to the adoption of different building procurement techniques by service providers, and flexible and innovative approaches are common. New relationships between clients, developers, architects and contractors are evolving and the roles and responsibilities of parties need to be fully understood. It is also important not to throw the baby out with the bath water. A poorly performing building is no bargain, however quickly and cheaply it was built; the enthusiastic adoption of fast-build package deal techniques has not always resulted in a satisfactory building, and good safeguards must be built into the systems to maintain quality.

3.2.1 Strategic planning

The core business of care home operators is the provision of residential beds, and although more care is being delivered to people in their own homes the demographic bias towards an increasing older population suggests there will be no reduction in the need for long-term residential care for the frail. Buildings are central to the strategic planning of the operators: they are the measure of their success, and the means by which the operation grows. Building acquisition, or the management of the building process is a key function.

The development role

Control of building projects may be the task of the director, chief executive or owner. Larger organizations may have a project manager in post, or buy in advice as required. The project manager may be an architect or other building professional. This role can be separate from the team appointed for a specific building project. It needs a creative and enterprising approach; the skills required are much more than the ability to control cost and time effectively, important though these are. Knowledge and understanding of both the building process and of the care profession are needed in areas such as:

- the objectives of the organisation and needs of its clients
- future directions in health care
- political, legal, social and commercial context
- finance, funding, and risk assessment
- property appraisal and space utilization
- development plans
- site selection and appraisal
- project team building
- briefing
- building procurement and contract law
- programming, monitoring, control of design, cost, quality and construction
- health and safety
- commissioning, staffing, operation, management and appraisal of buildings.

3.2.2 Building procurement

The options for providers are to build or to buy, or to do something in between. The choice of method is a matter of debate and judgement; each method has its advantages and disadvantages.

Traditional contract

The client appoints an architect to design and detail a building, and supervise the construction on site as described in the RIBA *Standard Form of Agreement for the Appointment of an Architect*. The architect co-ordinates the work of other building professionals, the quantity surveyor, structural and services engineers. Tenders are invited from contractors on the basis of production drawings and bills of quantities, and the successful contractor, usually the one with the lowest price, is appointed to carry out the work.

Advantages

- The client, through the architect keeps control of the project.
- The price is competitive on an equal basis.
- The relationships of the parties to the contract are unambiguous.
- There should be no conflict of interests.
- Good buildings can be produced by any method, properly controlled, but there is a commonly held view that buildings produced by traditional techniques are of higher quality with consistent detailing, better finishes and good landscaping.

Disadvantages	• The process is linear, i.e. virtually each section of work has to be completed before another can start, so it is the slowest method. • There is a lot of professional time (and fees) involved. • The actual building cost is not known until the project is a long way down the line.
Fast-track traditional	Techniques to offset some of the disadvantages of the traditional process are often adopted. Once a scheme design has been approved time and cost savings can be made in the pre- and post-contract periods The pre-contract process can be shortened if the client is prepared to risk fees for abortive work, and production information and bills of quantities are started before planning permission is obtained. The savings in interest charges will often justify taking calculated risks to move the start on site forward. Part of the works may be designed by the contractor, and thus taken off the critical path towards letting a contract. The Contractor's Design Portion Supplement to the JCT contract was evolved for this purpose. Contract periods can be shortened by the adoption of fast building techniques such as off-site manufacture, dry as opposed to wet systems, component building as a development of system building using readily available off-the-peg building parts.
Design and build	Design and build contracts are where the contractor does much and in some cases all of the design for a fixed lump sum. The contract is based on a set of employer's (client's) requirements and contractor's proposals and a contract sum analysis. The employer's requirements may be a simple schedule of accommodation or a detailed scheme design with specification. Clients may appoint an architect or quantity surveyor as an agent to assist in the preparation of the employer's requirements and to monitor the progress of the works. Architects may be novated to the contractor after the contract is signed, or may remain on the client's 'side' to perform a quality control and monitoring function, in which case contractors usually appoint their own architects to do the detailed building design. Contractors are either selected by a tendering process or appointed direct.
Advantages	• The project cost is known early. • Less parties are involved. • Contractors can use their buying power to obtain good prices. • The process is speedy. Bills of quantity are not required and production information does not have to be complete before site work commences.
Disadvantages	• Contractors can make large profits when they are not in price competition with each other. • Lack of detailed specification can result in poor building quality. • The client loses control over detailing, specification and finishes. Disputes are not easy to resolve. • The process is very dependant on the quality of the contractor. Clients, particularly the NHS Trusts who have used this procurement route report disappointing or patchy results. While there are successful projects there is also a high level of dissatisfaction. The cost certainty and time savings possible with design and build will always make it an attractive option. Skills in briefing and specification and contract control, and means of obtaining redress if things go wrong need to be given high priority.
Management contracts	There are many variations on the management contract theme. Broadly it is where the contractor is appointed early and is able to influence the design process. The contractor is paid a fee for input in the pre-construction stages and submits a tender for all or part of the building work. There is usually a

break clause in the middle. The contractor may take the lead role in managing the project or there may be another lead professional, an architect or surveyor. Construction works can be entirely the responsibility of the main contractor or smaller packages of work may be let to individual contractors, with the main contractor managing the interface and providing a general labour role to give continuity. Where a large number of small contracts are envisaged it may be appropriate to work to a budget rather than a fixed price This method is appropriate where there is a series of refurbishment works to be done, and is used for the upgrading of groups of former local authority homes. It may also be used for new build projects.

Advantages
- The contractor's expertise is available early so costly specifications and slow site processes can be eliminated.
- The process is speedy. Production information and bills of quantity do not necessarily have to be completed before site works commence.
- Critical components can be ordered in advance.

Disadvantages
- There may be no cost certainty until the end of the project.
- Cost competition is not guaranteed. Even where competitive tenders are obtained the appointed contractor has a considerable advantage, and it may be difficult and expensive to operate the break clause.

Turnkey contracts

The ultimate in minimizing exposure to risk is to buy a complete, fitted out and in some cases staffed-up building. New as well as existing buildings are acquired in this way. Reductions in capital spending programmes, particularly in the case of NHS Trusts are leading to partnerships with developers where the developer will finance, build, fit out and even staff-up a building in exchange for a guaranteed occupancy for a period of years. Contractual negotiations over future tenancy and fees can be difficult for both parties and are not always successful. It is a large risk for the developer to take.

Advantages
- Where the developer retains ownership no capital investment by the client (other than the site) is required.
- Risk is minimized.

Disadvantages
- There is loss of control by the user of building design.
- Refurbishment or alteration works may be needed. Where an existing building is purchased these can be extensive and are not always foreseen at the time of purchase.

Leasing

Capital costs can be significantly reduced by leasing parts of the building. Leasing arrangements are possible in an increasing number of fields. Some of the most common are:

- lift installation and other mechanical hoists
- fire alarm or nurse call systems
- kitchen and laundry
- furniture and fittings.

3.2.3 Briefing

A good brief is crucial to the success of a project, and especially so when innovative procurement methods are adopted. It is important that clear relationships are established at the beginning; it is surprising in practice how hard this can be to achieve. Briefing can seem a time-consuming and some-what tedious process but there is a high price to pay if it is not carried out thoroughly; it works much better when the client has a named individual or a forum set up for decision making. Information may include the following:

- a list of Health Authority or Local Authority Registration requirements
- schedule of accommodation
- room data sheets

Management of the building process

- external works data sheets
- building envelope
- furniture layouts
- room layouts (both plan and elevation may be appropriate in critical rooms, e.g. toilets for the disabled)
- services performance standards
- systems performance standards.

Examples of briefing documentation may be found in Technical Supplements 4–6.

3.2.4 Commissioning

Approvals

Approval in principle will be sought from the registering authority at the scheme design stage. It is important to keep up with changes in standards, as these are fairly frequently upgraded and may change between the scheme design stage and completion of the project.

Inspection

Before a building can be registered it must be inspected and approved by various officers. Co-ordination and organization of inspections needs to be a designated responsibility which can be taken by the client, the architect or the contractor. A check list of inspections and documentation which may be required is detailed in section 3.1.2.

Registration

A final inspection is made by the Registration Officer who then makes a recommendation to a committee who formally grant registration. In some cases the Registration Officer has delegated powers to register the building. Otherwise the recommendation has to be approved by the committee before the home can be occupied, so it is important to co-ordinate the building completion date with the committee cycle.

Technical supplements

114   TS1   List of suppliers

116   TS2   List of agencies concerned with older people

117   TS3   List of dangerous and poisonous plants

119   TS4   Initial briefing meeting agenda

120   TS5   Schedule of accommodation

122   TS6   Room data sheet

TS1 List of suppliers

Baths and hoists

Arjo Ltd
St Catherine's Street
Gloucester GL1 2SL
Tel. 01452 500200

Parker Bath Company Ltd
Queensway
Stem Lane
New Milton
Hampshire BH25 5NN
Tel. 01425 622287

Sluice

Caradon Twyfords Ltd
Twyfords Bathrooms
PO Box 23
Cliffe Vale
Stoke-on-Trent
Staffs ST4 7AL
Tel. 01270 879777

Stanbridge Ltd
32 Pope Road
Bromley
Kent BR2 9QB
Tel. 0181 464 0521

Dolphin Disinfection Company Ltd
14 Dawkins Road Industrial Estate
Hamworthy
Poole
Dorset BH15 4JY
Tel. 01202 667399

Clinical waste disposal

Cannon Hygiene Ltd
Middlegate
White Lund
Morecambe
Lancashire LA3 3BJ
Tel. 01524 60894

Waste disposal bins

Otto (UK) Ltd
Huntingdon Way
Measham
Swadlincote
Derbyshire D12 7DS
Tel. 01530 273939

Lifts

Evans Lifts Ltd
Abbey Lane
Leicester LE4 5QX
Tel. 01162 662464

Stannah Lifts Ltd
East Portway
Andover
Hants SP10 3LU
Tel. 01264 339090

Thyssen Lifts and Escalators Ltd
Traffic Street
Nottingham NG2 1NF
Tel. 01159 868213

Nurse call systems

Zettler UK
Zettler House
Pinner Road
Northwood
Middx HA6 1DL
Tel. 01923 826155

Ironmongery	HEWI (UK) Ltd	Josiah Parkes and Sons Ltd
	Scimitar Close	Helping Hand Hardware
	Gillingham Business Park	Union Works
	Gillingham	Gower Street
	Kent ME8 0RN	Willenhall
	Tel. 01634 377688	W. Midlands WV13 1JX
		Tel. 01902 366931

Threshold seals	Sealmaster Ltd
	Brewery Road
	Pampisford
	Cambridge CB2 4HG
	Tel. 01223 832851

Carpets	Birch International Carpets	Interface Europe Ltd (System Six)
	318 Coleford Road	The Gatehouse
	Darnall	Gatehouse Way
	Sheffield S9 5HP	Aylesbury
	Tel. 01142 435118	Bucks HP19 3DL
		Tel. 01296 393244

Age Concern England (ACE)
Bernard Sunley House
60 Pitcairn Road
Mitcham
Surrey, CR4 3LL

Arthritis and Rheumatism Council (ARC)
25 Bradiston Road
Maida Hill
London W9 3HN

British Association for Service to the Elderly
119 Hassell Street
Newcastle-under-Lyme
Staffs ST5 1AX

Centre for Accessible Environments
Nutmeg House
60 Gainsford Street
London SE1 2NY

Centre for Policy on Ageing
25–31 Ironmonger Row
London EC1V 3QP

DesignAge
Royal College of Art
Kensington Gore
London SW7 2EU

Helen Hamlyn Foundation
8 Bryanstone Mews East
London W1H 7FH

Help the Aged
16–18 St James's Walk
London EC1R 0BE

Horticultural Therapy
Goulds Ground
Vallis Way
Frome
Somerset BA11 3DW

Horticultural Trades Association
19 High Street
Theale
Reading
Berks RG7 5AH

The Relatives Association
5 Tavistock Place
London WC1H 9SS

Royal National Institute for the Deaf
105 Gower St
London WC1E 6AH

TS3 List of dangerous and poisonous plants

The following lists of dangerous plants are reproduced with permission from *The Horticultural Trades Association Code of Recommended Retail Practice Relating to the Labelling of Potentially Harmful Plants*, HTA (1994).

Category A The sale of these plants should be restricted and sales to the public discouraged. Display in retail areas should be supervised so that children do not have access. Individual plants should be labelled and customers should be informed of the potentially harmful nature of the plants by sales staff.

Rhus (only *R. radicans, R. succedanea, R. verniciflua*)	**CAUTION toxic if eaten; skin contact commonly causes severe blistering dermatitis**

Category B These plants require a warning on the plant label and on any bed label or any other point of sale material. The required warning text is indicated.

Aconitum	**CAUTION toxic if eaten**
Arum	**CAUTION toxic if eaten/skin + eye irritant**
Atropa	**CAUTION toxic if eaten**
Colchicum	**CAUTION toxic if eaten**
Convallaria majalis	**CAUTION toxic if eaten**
Daphne laureola	**CAUTION toxic if eaten/may cause skin allergy**
Daphne mezereum	**CAUTION toxic if eaten/may cause skin allergy**
Daphne (all other species)	**CAUTION toxic if eaten**
Datura	**CAUTION toxic if eaten**
Dictamnus albus	**CAUTION skin irritant in sunlight**
Dieffenbachia	**CAUTION toxic if eaten/skin + eye irritant**
Digitalis	**CAUTION toxic if eaten**
Gaultheria (section *Pernettya* only)	**CAUTION toxic if eaten**
Gloriosa superba	**CAUTION toxic if eaten**
Hyoscyamus	**CAUTION toxic if eaten**
Laburnum	**CAUTION toxic if eaten**
Lantara	**CAUTION toxic if eaten**
Nerium oleander	**CAUTION toxic if eaten**
Phytolacca	**CAUTION toxic if eaten**
Primula obconica	**CAUTION may cause skin allergy**
Ricinus communis	**CAUTION toxic if eaten**
Ruta	**CAUTION severely toxic to skin in sunlight**
Solanum dulcamara	**CAUTION toxic if eaten**
Taxus	**CAUTION toxic if eaten**
Veratrum	**CAUTION toxic if eaten**

Category C These plants require a warning label. The required warning text is indicated.

Aesculus	**Harmful if eaten**
Agrostemma githago	**Harmful if eaten**
Alstroemeria	**May cause skin allergy**
Aquilegia	**Harmful if eaten**
Brugmansia	**Harmful if eaten**
Caltha	**Harmful if eaten**
Catharanthus roseus	**Harmful if eaten**
Cupressocyparis leylandii	**May cause skin allergy**
Delphinium	**Harmful if eaten**
Dendranthema (formerly *Chrysanthemum*) (excluding pot mums)	**May cause skin allergy**
Echium	**Skin irritant**

Euonymus	**Harmful if eaten**
Euphorbia (except *E. pulcherrima*, Poinsettia)	**Harmful if eaten/skin + eye irritant**
Ficus carica	**Skin irritant in sunlight**
Fremontodendron	**Skin + eye irritant**
Gaultheria (except section *Pernettya*)	**Harmful if eaten**
Hedera	**Harmful if eaten/may cause skin allergy**
Helleborus	**Harmful if eaten**
Hyacinthus (except planted bowls)	**Skin irritant**
Hypericum perforatum	**Harmful if eaten**
Ipomoea	**Harmful if eaten**
Iris	**Harmful if eaten**
Juniperus sabina (except exclusively juvenile forms)	**Harmful if eaten**
Kalmia	**Harmful if eaten**
Ligustrum	**Harmful if eaten**
Lobelia tupa	**Harmful if eaten/skin + eye irritant**
Lupinus	**Harmful if eaten**
Narcissus (except planted bowls)	**Harmful if eaten/skin irritant**
Ornithogalum	**Harmful if eaten**
Polygonatum	**Harmful if eaten**
Prunus laurocerasus	**Harmful if eaten**
Rhamnus	**Harmful if eaten**
Schefflera	**May cause skin allergy**
Scilla	**Harmful if eaten**
Thuja	**Harmful if eaten**
Tulipa (except planted bowls)	**Skin irritant**
Wisteria	**Harmful if eaten**

TS4   Initial briefing meeting agenda

Project

name   number   size and description

Budget   **Appointment and scope of service**

Site
address

telephone
fax
ownership

Client
name
address

telephone
fax

Client's named representative	**Briefing team**	**Manager or Matron**
name		name
address		address
telephone		telephone
fax		fax

Registration Authority	**Planning Authority**	**Building Control**
name	name	name
address	address	address
telephone	telephone	telephone
fax	fax	fax

Programme
design proposals
approvals:
planning
building regulations
registration Authority
other statutory authorities
start on site
completion

TS5 Schedule of accommodation

	Space	No.	Dimensions
Circulation	Circulation spaces		
	Reception		
	Entrance areas		
	Lifts		
	Lift motor rooms		
Residents' living areas	Bedsitting rooms		
	En-suite toilets		
	Guest bedrooms		
	Close care flats		
	Day areas		
	Hairdressing		
	Dining areas		
	Kitchenettes		
Residents' ablutions	Bathing		
	Residents' toilets		
Residents' care	Nurse station		
	Sluice, dirty utility		
	Treatment, clean utility		
	Drug store		
Storage	Linen		
	Wheelchairs		
	Equipment		
	Long term		
	Continence aids		
	Cleaning equipment		
Administration	Administration office		
	Manager/matron's office		
	Staff rooms		
	Staff cloaks		
	Staff toilet		
	Shower		
	Visitors' toilets		

Technical supplements

	Space	No.	Dimensions
Kitchen and laundry	Kitchen		
	Kitchen stores		
	Wash up		
	Vegetable preparation		
	Meal preparation		
	Staff toilet		
	Laundry		
External spaces	Vehicle and pedestrian access		
	Service yard		
	Garden		

Additional requirements

TS6 Room data sheet

Page: Project: Block:

Room name/number :   Drawing no: Agreed by/signed:

Area: Date:

		ref.	size	quantity	group
Elements	Door				
	Ironmongery				
	Window				
	Ironmongery				
Finishes	Floor				
	Ceiling				
	Walls				
	Door				
	Windows				
	Woodwork				
Services	Heating/temperature				
	Lighting, day				
	Lighting, artificial				
	Power				
	Shaver point				
	Nurse call				
	Telephone				
	Television				
	Security				
	Monitor				
	Ventilation				
	Hot water				
	Cold water				
	Drainage				

Fittings and fixtures

Further reading

Statutory requirements and recommended standards are also listed on pp. 103–107.

British Gypsum (1991) *The White Book*. Loughborough, British Gypsum Ltd.

British Standards Institute (1980) *BS 5906:1980 Code of Practice for Storage and Onsite Treatment of Solid Waste from Buildings*. Milton Keynes, BSI.

British Standards Institute (1986) *BS 1415 Part 2:19 Whole Body Immersion Fail Safe Thermostatic Devices*. Milton Keynes, BSI.

British Standards Institute (1991) *BS 4467:1991 Guide to Dimensions in Designing for Elderly People*. Milton Keynes, BSI.

British Standards Institute (1993) *BS 7594:1993 The Code of Practice of Audio Frequency Induction Loop Systems*. Milton Keynes, BSI.

Brundett, G.W.B. (1992) *Legionella and Building Services*. Oxford, Butterworth Heinemann.

Centre for Policy on Ageing (1984) *Home Life: A code of practice for residential care*. London, CPA.

CPA (1996) *A Better Home Life*. London, CPA.

CIBSE (1994) *Code for Interior Lighting*. London, CIBSE.

Department of Environment/Welsh Office (1991) *Building Regulations. Approved document B*. London, HMSO.

Department of Health and Social Security (1987) *Firecode. HTM 81 Fire precautions in new hospitals*. London, HMSO. (These guidelines can be used for residential homes.)

Department of Health and Social Security (1989) *Firecode. Nucleus fire precautions recommendations*. London, HMSO.

Department of Health and Social Security (1990) *Caring for Quality: guidance on standards for residential homes for elderly people*. London, HMSO.

Department of Health and Social Security (1991) *Code of Practice. Control of Legionellae in health care premises* (and amendments 1 and 2). London, HMSO.

Goldsmith, S. (1976) *Designing for the Disabled.* London, RIBA Publications.

Health and Safety Executive (1991) *Approved code of practice – the prevention or control of legionellosis (including Legionnaire's disease).* London, HMSO.

HMSO (1992) *Long-term Care for Elderly People; purchasing, providing and quality.* London, HMSO.

Hollingbery, R. (1993) *Multipurpose Centres for Elderly People.* London, The Helen Hamlyn Foundation.

Home Office (1982) *Draft Guide to Fire Precautions in Existing Hospitals.* London, Home Office.

Home Office/Scottish Home and Health Department (1983) *Draft Guide to Fire Precautions in Existing Residential Care Premises.* London, Home Office. (This guide can be used for new as well as existing buildings.)

Marshall, M. (1992) Designing for Disorientation. *Access by Design,* (May/August), 15–17.

National Association of Health Authorities and Trusts (1985, 1988 supplement) *Registration and Inspection of Nursing Homes: a handbook for health authorities.* Birmingham, NAHAT.

National Federation of Housing Associations (1993) *Accommodation Diversity: the design of housing for minority ethnic, religious and cultural groups.* London, NFHA.

Salmon, G. (1993) *Caring Environments for Frail Elderly People.* London, Longman.

Valins, M. (1988) *Housing for Elderly People: a guide for architects and clients.* London, Butterworth.

Willcocks, D., Pearce, S. and Kellaher, L. (1987) *Private Lives in Public Places.* London, Tavistock Publications.

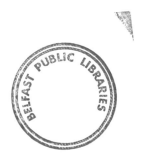

Further reading

Index

Page numbers appearing in **bold** refer to Figures, and numbers in *italics* refer to Tables.

Access 7
  building layout 7
  gardens 97
  pedestrian 96
  ramps 7, 96
  registration
    requirements 104
  vehicle 93
Acoustics 9, 79
Administration 70
Ageing process 4
Agencies 116
Alarm call, *see* Nurse
call
Alzheimer's disease 12
Ambulift **60**
Anthropometric data **35**
Apartments 41, 46
Approvals 103
  checklist 107
Arthritis 9
Attitudes to old age 2
Audio-frequency
induction loops 80

Bathroom fittings,
fixing heights **57**
Bathrooms 55
  access dimensions
    56
  building elements 62
  environment 62
  finishes 55
  fittings 55
  furniture 61
  services 61
  user requirements
    55
Baths, specialist **58, 59**
  dimensions **58**
Bed-sitting rooms 41
Bedroom furniture,

dimensions **44**
Bedrooms 41
  building elements 43
  environment 42
  finishes 42
  fittings 42
  furniture 42, **44**
  services 42
  user requirements
    42
  window cill height
    45
Beds, dimensions **43**
Bin store **97**
Brief 110
  briefing meeting
    agenda *119*
British Standards 123
Building Control
Officer 30, 107
Building layout
considerations
  dementia 23
  day care 33
  ethnic groups 24
  incontinence 11
  mobility 7
  staff 29
  visitors 31
Building procurement
108

Car parking 96
  wheelchair parking
    96
Care staff 27
Chairs **49**
Circulation spaces 36
  building elements 36
  critical dimensions
    37
  environment 36

finishes 36
fittings 36
services 36
user requirements
  36
Clean utility 66
Cleaner's store 70
Cloakroom, staff 73
Close care flats 46
Codes of practice 106
Colour 77
  colour vision 9
  dementia 21
  landscape, planting
    98
Commissioning 111
Community
Pharmacist 30, 107
Contract
  design and build 109
  fast track 109
  management 109
  traditional 108
  turnkey 110
Controls 82
Corridors 36

Day areas 47
  building elements
    49
  environment 49
  finishes 48
  fittings 48
  furniture 48
  services 48
  user requirements
    47
Day care 33
Dayrooms, *see* Day
areas
Deafness 9, 79
Decoration 22, 78

Dementia 11–23
    design for 15
    environmental
    design 21
    garden design 22
    key points 23
    nature of 12
    reinforcement of
    reality 20
    statistics 12
Design and build 109
Dining 51
    building elements 52
    environment 52
    finishes 51
    furniture 51
    services 52
    user requirements
    51
Dining tables
    circulation space **52**
    dimensions **53**
    heights and thigh
    clearances **51**
Dirty utility 65
Domus 17
Drug store 66

Electrics 82
Elevator, *see* Lifts
Emergency power 85
Entrances 38
    environment 39
    finishes 38
    fittings 39
    furniture 39
    services 39
    user requirements
    38
Entryphone 86
Environmental Health
Officer 30, 107
Ethnic minority groups
23–25
Eyesight 8
External works, *see*
Landscape

Fast track 109
Fire Officer 30, 107
Fire prevention 86–7
    alarms 86
    emergency lighting
    87
    flame retardent
    materials 87
    means of escape 87
Flats 46

Gardens 97–102

Glare 9, 77
Guest rooms 43

Hairdresser 33
Hairdressing 49
Handrail dimensions **37**
Health And Safety At
Work Act 1974
    staff
    accommodation 28
Hearing 9, 79
Heating 81
Helen Hamlyn
Foundation 33
Hoists **60**

Incontinence 10
Inspection Officers 29,
103
    Nursing Homes 29
    Residential Homes
    30
Inspections 107
Insurance certificates
107
Interior design 77

Kitchen 74
    environment 75
    finishes 74
    fittings 74
    services 74
    user requirements
    74
Kitchenettes 54

Landscape 90–102
    external lighting 101
    seating **101**
    tables **102**
Landscape design,
ethnic minority
groups 25
Laundry 75
    finishes 76
    fittings 76
    services 76
    user requirements
    75
Lay Assessors 30
Leasing 110
Legionnaires'
disease 84
Legislation 106
Lifting aids **60**
Lifts
    dimensions,
    8-person hydraulic
    lift **40**
    environment 41

finishes 41
fittings 41
lighting 41
services 41
user requirements
39
Light 77
Lightening conductor
84
Lighting 8, 77
    external 101
Linen store, *see*
Storage
Living rooms, *see* Day
areas
Local Authority homes
25
Location, *see* Site
location
Lounges, *see* Day areas

Madison bath **58, 59**
Management
    building process 107
    home management
    26
Management structure
27
Manager 26
Manual dexterity 9
Matron 26
Means of escape, *see*
Fire prevention
Mobility 5, 7
Monitored line 86

NHS homes 25
NHS Trust Homes 25
Novaturn Taps **61**
Nurse call 87
    confused residents
    90
    call point mounting
    heights **88**
    linked
    communications *89,*
    90
    location *89*
    system controls *89*
Nurse station 64

Office 70
Osteoporosis 5
Overnight stay 43
Owners 25

Parker bath **58, 59**
Parkinson's disease 9
Part Three homes 25
Pharmacist 30, 107

Planning Officer 30, 107
Planning restrictions,
space between
buildings **94**
Planting 99
Plants
    poisonous 101
    poisonous, list of
    117
Population statistics 1
Power 82
Private homes 25
Progressive Privacy 33
Project management
107
Providers of care 25

Radiators, surface
temperatures 82
Raised beds **100**
Refuse bins,
dimensions **97**
Refuse collection 96
Registered Homes Act
103, 106
Registration 103
    guidelines 103
    summary of
    requirements 104
Regulations 106
Relations 30
Relatives 30
Residents' toilets 62
    dimensions **63**
Respite care 34
Restaurant, *see* Dining
Road junctions **95**
Room data sheet *122*
Room temperatures
82

Sanitary fittings, *see*
Bathroom fittings
Schedule of
accommodation *120*
Seating **49**
Security 85
Self closing doors 4, 86
Service yard 97
Services
    electrics 82
    emergency power 85
    heating and

ventilation 81
telephone 84
water 84
Shower, staff 73
Signs 79
    design **79**
    position of **79**
Site location 90
Slop hopper and sink
dimensions 65
Sluice 65
    automatic **65**
Socket heights **83**
Sound insulation 80
Sound reduction
targets *81*
Staff
    accommodation 28,
    73
    care assistants 27
    domestic 29
    manager 26
    matron 26
    rooms 72
    toilets 73
Standards 106
Statistics 1
Statutory requirements
106
Storage
    cleaning equipment
    70
    continence aids 69
    equipment 68
    linen 67
    long term 69
    wheelchairs 68
    wheelchair
    dimensions **68**
Suppliers *114*
Switches 83
    heights **83**
    selection **83**
Systems
    fire prevention 86
    nurse call 87
    security 85

Table heights 51
    see also Dining
    tables
Taps 10, **61**
Telephone 84

induction couplers
80
Television 84
Temperatures, room
82
Thermostats
    heating 82
    hot water 84
Thresholds 8
Toilets 62
    dimensions **63**
    finishes 62
    fittings 62
    kitchen staff 74
    services 63–4
    staff 73
    user requirements
    62
    visitors 71
Toilets, assisted
dimensions **64**
Treatment room 66

Vehicle access 93
Ventilation 82
Visibility splay **95**
Vision
    visual performance 8
    perception 77
Visitors
    checklist of
    requirements 31
    community 31
    day care 33
    hairdresser 33
    personal 30
    professional 31
    respite care 34
Voluntary homes 25

W.C., *see* Toilets
Washing machines 76
Water 84
Water temperatures 84
Wheelchairs
    dimensions **35**
    parking bays **96**
    storage 68
    turning space in
    bathroom **56**
    turning space in
    bedroom **43**
Window cill height **45**